OLIVE OIL

OLIVE OIL

The Good Heart Protector

Rita Greer and Cyril Blau

SOUVENIR PRESS

First published 1995 by Souvenir Press Ltd,
43 Great Russell Street, London WC1B 3PA
and simultaneously in Canada

ISBN 0 285 63237 X

Photoset by Rowland Phototypesetting Ltd
Bury St Edmunds, Suffolk
Printed in Great Britain by
The Guernsey Press Co. Ltd., Guernsey, Channel Islands.

Contents

Acknowledgements

The authors would like to thank the following for their help in researching this book:

London: Sternberg Centre for Jewish Learning; A. S. Ashaad, Muslim Welfare Centre; Charles Carey, The Oil Merchant; The British Library; Italian Embassy and Trade Centre; Winecellars, Wandsworth; Sotheby's Auction House; Christie's Auction House; Michael and Jaqueline Mina; Dr Robert Woodward; the Real Food Store, Little Venice. Liane McNabb (French translation).

Southern England: Kew Gardens, Richmond; Blagden Chemicals; Martin MacKenzie-Smith, Senior Chemist, Hampshire Cosmetics Ltd; the Rev. Derek Mottershead, St Xaviour's Church, Eastbourne.

Athens: Archaeological Museum; Maria and Tassos Strofalis.

MAIL ORDER COMPANIES

Kitchen equipment, including oil drizzlers, Lakeland Plastics Ltd., Alexandra Buildings, Windermere, Cumbria LA23 1BQ.
Olive oil, The Oil Merchant, 47, Ashworth Grove, London W12 9BU.

AUTHOR'S NOTE

Every effort has been made to trace the owners of any copyright material quoted in this book in order to seek the necessary permission. Where these efforts have proved unsuccessful, the authors will be glad to hear from copyright owners so that appropriate acknowledgement can be made in any subsequent reprint.

CHAPTER 1

Olive to Oil

With so many cooking oils on the market from which to choose, at competitive prices, why is olive oil, the most expensive, becoming so popular? It has been around for thousands of years so there can hardly be anything new about it. The answer is partly the shift in attitude by the consumer, which has come about for a variety of reasons, and, most important, a new interest in healthy eating.

Good health is something to be valued—beyond price. It is influenced by many factors such as geographical location, climate, race, lifestyle, physical fitness, occupation, inherited health factors, age, build, affluence and diet. Some illnesses are inherited with our genes: disorders that 'run in the family' are passed down generation to generation, every other generation or down either the male or female line. Others are illnesses to which people are predisposed—in other words, they might occur if given the appropriate circumstances. Many are brought on and made irreversible by lifestyle, particularly smoking and poor diet. The bad habits of a lifetime can lead to constant ill health or a crisis, involving obesity, diabetes, gout, chronic constipation, diverticulitis, strokes and heart attacks. Most of this misery could be avoided if people lived and ate in a more sensible way.

As research goes on into diet, heart and circulation, more evidence is being put forward to show that olive oil can protect the blood and heart. In Greece and Italy the incidence of heart disease is at least five times lower than in the UK, and although the Italians and Greeks eat double the amount of vegetables that we do, they also consume more fat. Scientists have put this down to the fact that the staple fat of both countries is olive oil, whereas in the UK it is not.

What does olive oil contain to make it not merely harmless, but actively beneficial to health? Scientists are still working on this, but their researches have so far indicated that olive oil in the diet can help us in a number of ways.

Cholesterol
Cholesterol, which has a bad name in modern health folklore, is in fact an important substance needed for healthy cells and hormones (it is not actually a fat but a fat-like lipid). The liver needs fat to help make the necessary cholesterol but too much fat intake can lead to too much cholesterol production. (Gallstones, which can form in the gallbladder, are a solid form of cholesterol.) A build-up of cholesterol in the artery walls reduces the diameter of the channel used by the blood to transport nutrients around the body. More pressure is required to force the blood through, which interferes with its free flow. Problems arise and the real crisis is a heart attack, stroke or blood clots.

Cholesterol is transported around the body in the bloodstream with the help of lipoproteins—high density lipoproteins (HDLs) and low density lipoproteins (LDLs). LDLs are not as useful as HDLs because they clog up the artery walls with cholesterol deposits. Olive oil, due to its high level of monounsaturates, seems to be able to raise the number of HDLs in the blood while lowering the LDLs, keeping the cholesterol level down. It is now known that saturated and animal fats increase the level of harmful LDLs and too much polyunsaturated fat can lower the beneficial HDLs.

Circulation

In a trial at a London hospital, 1½ tablespoons of olive oil were taken daily by volunteers. When their blood was examined it could be seen that the platelets had been discouraged from clumping together, lessening the risk of clots and strokes. This was due to a fatty acid in the olive oil. Circulation is made easier if the artery walls are fairly elastic, allowing them to expand. It is thought olive oil may be able to achieve this, making circulation of the blood easier and blood pressure lower.

Antioxidants

The natural antioxidants present in olive oil help to prevent rancidity. These can be of benefit in the body as they help to fight off the damaged cells (free radicals) which can cause the arteries to clog, overload the immune system and, it is thought, contribute to the growth of cancer cells.

Healing

Olive oil is known to have healing properties. The relation-ship between the ingestion of olive oil and a reduction in gastric fluid concentration has been the subject of several studies. When olive oil is substituted for animal fats in the diet the result can be a decline in stomach ulcers. Olive oil can have an effect on gastric lesions, as in gastro-duodenal ulcers, described as a 'protective therapeutic effect'.

Gallstones

By clearing a chemical from the liver olive oil can help detoxify the body. Dietary management of gallstones is possible with olive oil as it is thought to contain the ideal proportions of fatty acids for the purpose.

11

Growth and Prevention

Experiments have shown that development of cerebral tissue in babies is superior where the babies are fed on mother's milk when the mother's diet contains olive oil. Diabetes and atherosclerosis can be prevented by a diet which includes olive oil. There is ample evidence to support this as there have been many successful trials.

With all these scientifically proven benefits, is it any wonder that olive oil is now rated so highly in the health stakes? However, if you want to get the most out of this oil you need to know how to use it sensibly in your diet. Taken in moderation, as part of an overall eating plan, it will undoubtedly improve your health, and you will begin to understand why the olive has attracted so much mythology and folklore in the countries where it has been a staple part of the diet and a way of life for thousands of years.

*   *   *

It is hard to imagine Mediterranean countries before the olive was cultivated there. Now it is typical of the landscape: deep blue sea, a cloudless sky, rocky hills, fertile plains—and olive trees. In Italy alone there are more than 1,200,000 hectares of olive groves, mostly on hilly ground that would not be used for any other crop. Some 26 centuries have passed since the first cultivated olive shoots were grafted on to the wild olive, and today Italy sustains a huge industry, importing olives for oil production from other countries to add to its own enormous harvest.

Figures from the Italian Trade Centre in London gave an insight into the scale of world production. The EC produces over 1,300,000 tonnes of olive oil every year, the largest tonnages coming from Spain, Italy and Greece, with much smaller quantities from Portugal and France. France, Portugal and Italy consume more than they produce, so Spain and Greece have a market for their excess production on the doorstep, but 130,000 tonnes are also exported annually to other parts of the world, mainly the USA and Libya. Outside the EC there is substantial olive oil production in other countries bordering the Mediterranean—Tunisia, Morocco, Algeria, Turkey and Syria.

CULTIVATION AND HARVESTING

The olive tree, *Olea europaea*, was one of the first known cultivated trees. It is an evergreen and grows around the world largely between 30°–45° North and 30°–45° South. The Mediterranean type of climate is ideal for growth, propagation and harvest and, by no coincidence, the olive grows where the vine flourishes. Long sunny summers, light spring and winter rains and rarely any frost provide ideal conditions.

The trees grow slowly and reach a height of three to ten metres. They have many small branches which bear lance-shaped leathery leaves, sage green or dark green on top with a silvery underside. The trunks are dark greyish and brown and are often gnarled and twisted. They can grow and bear fruit for centuries, and take between four and eight years to reach the stage of producing the first olive fruits, often taking up to 20 years to produce a full crop. Some years they have a rest and produce no fruit at all.

Propagation
Growing from seed is not a popular method of propagation as it does not produce the best olives. The buds of the olive tree are unusual in that they are on the axil of each leaf and on the roots themselves. This enables cuttings to be taken from the tree.

Because olive trees grow for centuries, there is not a

Branch with ripening olives.

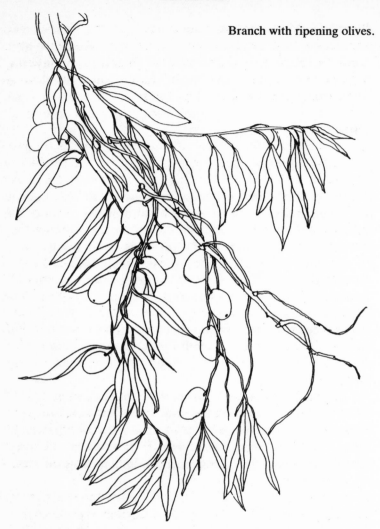

great deal of cutting down and replanting of trees, but much argument goes on about the best way to propagate in order to produce fertile types that will bear fruit for generations to come. Some old methods of propagation definitely do not produce good trees. A branch split into four at the base, with an olive stone planted in each one, leads to hollow-trunked trees. Using suckers and layering are also not always successful and taking too many cuttings can damage otherwise healthy trees.

Olive Groves

Groves are usually planted out in orderly rows of trees which are all about the same age. The silvery undersides of the leaves make them seem luminescent; at night they have a ghostly appearance. It is no surprise that in old religions they were worshipped as sacred goddesses. The foliage has an almost tousled look and if there are many branches they can appear almost matted, so prolific are the leaves.

The scale of the trees seems much more related to man than the tall trees we enjoy in wetter climates. In a well-kept olive grove there is a feeling of an age-old peace. The old, gnarled trunks and silvery crowns of foliage will have withstood the ravages of time—countless hot summers and mild winters, spring flowerings and harvests.

Damage

Severe gales can sometimes cause damage, snapping off branches and boughs that have taken many years to grow, and a cold spell with hard frosts can do untold damage. Generally, however, the life force of the tree is exceptionally strong and even trees struck by lightning will begin to grow again.

In 1985 the writer Piero Antolini endured the experience of seeing severe frost damage to both vines and olive trees. He journeyed through Italy by car along Highway 222, between Florence and Sienna, and found it distressing:

> . . . olives with leafless branches outstretched like the fingers of skeletons above blasted trunks, oozing

ruddy sap, or others in their orderly rows with silvery foliage whose luminescence has been darkened by clusters of leaves that had been stricken, dried out and sterilised by blasts of glacial winds but that were still attached, along with those still healthy, to fearless survivors.

He was shocked at the devastation, the injured and tormented trees and the change in the landscape, but cheered by young, single olive trees which gave him the impression they would regain life and fecundity. If the frosts had been even more severe, none of the trees would have survived in Chianti country—a chilling tragedy.

Fruit
Botanically the olive fruit is similar to the peach or plum, with a central stone containing the seed, fleshy covering and skin. There are many varieties of *Olea europaea*, most suited for oil, the rest for the table. The olive fruit is oval and about the size of a large damson. After wind pollination the small white spring flowers develop into green fruits which swell and ripen, and by October or November the first fruit is ripe. Some varieties are left on the tree and turn through green to purple to black. These are often left whole for pickling and serving at the table and account for ten per cent of olive production. Their bitter flavour is neutralised by soaking in brine for several weeks. Great skill is required in choosing the time to harvest.

Harvesting
One of the reasons why olive oil commands a high price is its labour-intensive harvesting. The fruit, being small, is easily contaminated by soil and ferments quickly when taken off the trees. By shaking or beating the tree with sticks or poles, the ripe olives will fall onto nets or cloths

spread underneath. This is called 'harvesting by natural fall'. Although the trees are tough and resilient, the shaking or beating can sometimes injure fruit-bearing branches and make them susceptible to bacterial disease. From a producer's point of view, however, the damage done is balanced against the 20–30 per cent extra oil which can be obtained from olives whose skin has darkened and for which this method is appropriate.

Hand picking, although expensive, is still the best method, as the fruit will be unbruised and the tree undamaged, and about 20 per cent of Italian olive oil is still derived from hand-picked olives. The best area for olive oil is Lucca which sustains a large industry, although not necessarily from olives grown in that area. Hand picking is used for the highest quality oils and is laborious, to say the least.

Where natural fall is used for harvesting, the olives must not be left on the nets for more than 15 days before collection. A good deal of hard labour is still involved in this method, and Californian growers are now beginning to use mechanical shakers. However, this presents problems because of the strong attachment between the fruit and the tree and because the trees are unable to stand the vibration.

MAKING THE OIL

After harvesting, by whatever means, extraction of the oil must follow as soon as possible. Domestic growers take their crops to the communal press for more or less immediate extraction. Villagers tend to give the press a wide berth at this time, as the smell of the newly crushed olives is pungent and unpleasant.

For the large producer a short period of storage is inevitable. This is a difficult time as chemical changes may occur which can lead to deterioration. Fermentation of the olives by enzymes naturally present in the fruit tissues, bacteria, yeasts and moulds, are all a risk during this waiting time. The olives must not be stored piled up as this encourages deterioration. With every farm bringing in its harvest around the same time, immediate pressing is not possible and queues form. Cool or refrigerated rooms for storage at the oil press would be an asset.

Traditional Milling
Once the olives have been transported to the press, the task is to extract the oil and bottle it for marketing. There is a certain cachet in using the traditional method of crushing the olives with stone mills and extracting the oil by pressure. This used to be done with animal or manpower but nowadays is done by electricity. The olives are picked over and washed only once. The grinding wheels are usually granite and it takes about an hour to crush the fruit, with the stones included in the crushing. The resulting paste is placed on esparto grass or synthetic mats, one on top of the other on a vertical pole, under a hydraulic press. Slowly the pressure is increased and the precious oil is squeezed out. A centrifuge filters the oil and removes the water from the paste. Sludgy water emerges from one pipe and oil from the other.

Traditionalists maintain this old method of pressing is the best. Although it is much slower than more modern methods and requires more manpower, the fresh, delicate flavours of the oil are more likely to be preserved and the method is definitely 'cold'.

Modern Extraction
Modern methods are slightly different but achieve the same end. The advantages are less handling of the olives and faster production on an automated system. Centri-

18

fuges and hydraulic presses are used in a series of processes and it is more hygienic.

The first process is to wash the olives (up to four times) and remove earth, leaves, twigs and any foreign bodies. This ensures a better-tasting oil, unlikely to be bitter. Next the olives are crushed and made into paste with a series of stainless steel blades. The result is a mixture of oil and water and solid pulp and pips. This is moved to a stainless steel chamber, and at a temperature of about 30°C the oil is extracted by centrifuge. More centrifugation is required to separate the oil from the water. Both emerge from the centrifuge warm.

You can see how the traditionalists using the true cold pressing method will disagree with the more modern methods. Obviously they are never going to agree over it. There is a great deal of old machinery about and not all of it is stainless steel, nor are all the pressing mats daisy fresh. The old methods are slow and expensive; the newer methods are faster and more hygienic. By coincidence they both produce good and not so good olive oils.

Storage

The oil is stored in big terracotta jars or stainless steel containers until ready for bottling. Unfiltered oil looks murky and unattractive, due to its sediment. This can be removed in the settling or filtering processes. Natural settling, when the oil comes to the top and the water goes to the bottom, is used by some producers, and filtering through cotton or synthetic cloths is preferred by others.

The third type of pressing requires heat and chemical treatment, as any oil left in the pomace (residue) is, by now, difficult to extract. Chemical methods are destructive of the natural nutrients of the oil, so sometimes these are added to this type of refined olive oil to try to restore its nutritional quality, for example vitamin E. Other factors which the processing changes are the colour and the aroma.

Oils that are to be used commercially for margarine and mayonnaise (which are stored at low temperatures) are cooled to just above freezing for 30 hours to allow crystallisation of high melting point glycerides. They are then filtered out.

Best Quality Culinary Olive Oils
The more slowly the olives ripen the lower the acidity of the oil produced from them, with the best oils not exceeding ½ per cent. Usually a green, spicy oil indicates a low acidity and the gentler yellow oils a higher acidity. Two important factors are the altitude at which the olives are grown, and the latitude. Groves in the coolest areas within the growing area usually produce the best oils. Variety of olive can also affect the acidity level, and quick crushing helps to keep the level of acidity low. All processes are designed to make the best quality oil possible, but the wait between harvesting and processing can lower the quality of oil produced.

By-Products
All kinds of processing can take place to extract olive oil by-products from the pomace. These are used in the manufacture of soaps, shampoos, conditioners, cosmetics, preparations and toiletries and are usually made from the lower grade refined oils.

Adulteration
The fact that olive oil can be processed and treated with chemicals and still look like olive oil leaves it wide open to adulteration. Although the two best grades of unrefined, unadulterated oil are the most costly, the aroma and taste still need to be acceptable. Sometimes they are blended off

to improve them or other lower grade oils. Results can be mysterious.

Varieties

It is difficult to put a number to the varieties of olive grown. Estimates vary from around forty to hundreds. Some growers have rows of different varieties in their groves in order to blend their oils for the market. Some oils start off with a particular flavour and then after storage develop another. A few months later they can revert more or less to the original flavour. Here is where the blending technique is essential to correct flavour. Using up an olive oil soon after you buy it would seem to be a good policy as the flavour could change with time.

Names of the varieties are influenced by the area where the olives are grown and the family who grew them centuries ago. For instance, the Ornelliaia estate in Italy has groves of mainly Frantoio and Moraiolo, with a few Leccino to give weight to the blend. The average age of the olive trees on the estate is about eighty years and there are no plans to introduce any other varieties of tree.

The oil from each harvest will be different from the previous year and varying amounts will be produced. Colour will vary, also taste and aroma. There are good years and bad years, as with all harvests.

GRADING OF OLIVE OIL FOR THE MARKET

Tasting

Within the EC, which is where most of the world's olives are grown, tasting panels and chemical analysis are used for official grading of olive oils. Custom-built testing rooms with individual booths are used by up to ten trained people entrusted with the tasting. The tasters do not sample more than five oils at any one sitting, and to ensure that the tasters are not influenced by the colour of the oils, they are served in blue glasses.

There are two classes of Virgin Oil which are obtained by mechanical or physical processes and have undergone only washing, decantation, centrifugation and filtration without heat treatment. No use of solvents, re-esterification processes or mixing with other oils is allowed for these two top-class olive oils.

The difference between them is in their acidity and the order of pressing. The acidity of Extra Virgin Olive Oil (first pressing) must not exceed 1 per cent (expressed as oleic acid. Virgin Olive Oil (second pressing), must not exceed 2 per cent. The lower quality oils produced by these two pressings with acidity levels too high are Common (not exceeding 3.3 per cent) and Clear Virgin (over 3.3 per cent) olive oil. Common Virgin Olive Oil has a good taste, Clear has an imperfect taste.

By refining the Common and Clear Virgin Oils, oils with a 0.5 per cent (or less) acidity level can be made. These can be blended with other refined and non-refined virgin olive oils, producing an oil with less than 1.5 per cent acidity. Oil of Olive Husks (Husk Oil) can be made by treatment with solvents, refining and blending for use in industry. The grades are Crude Olive Oil, refined Olive Oil and just Olive Oil.

In the United States, different names apply to grades. Best quality is 'Virgin', unrefined olive oil from the first pressing; 'Fine' quality usually means unrefined and re-fined blended together, although it may also be labelled 'Sansa and Olive oil.'

All grades of oil produced are used. Extra Virgin and Virgin are for best culinary use, especially salads. Pure olive oil is a lower grade for frying. The remaining grades are used for cosmetics and industry. Somehow every harvest gets used up due to demand. There's no olive oil lake—turnover is quick, almost relentless—and the culinary market is growing steadily as health becomes a more important factor in the Western diet.

Grades on Sale
In shops, Extra Virgin, Virgin and Olive Oil or Pure Olive Oil are on sale. Fino is another name sometimes used on Virgin Olive Oil. Light or Fine are two new, cheaper additions to the range of refined oil. Although gourmets and purists will throw up their hands in horror, a sobering thought is that if we all used Extra Virgin Olive Oil, there wouldn't be enough to go round.

The oil is packed and sold in tins, glass bottles or special plastic bottles and must be stored out of the light to prevent oxidisation.

NEW VINTAGES

On the single estates and in villages, the new season's olive oils are tasted: there are celebration meals and festivals for the results of the new harvest. In the UK, at the oil merchants', the new oils are greeted with as much enthusiasm and excitement as Beaujolais Nouveau. Here is a typical example from tasting notes for the 1993 harvest for the Allegrini estate in Italy.

Allegrini
Location: the hills of Valpolicella Classico, north-west of Verona. The proximity of Lake Garda moderates the climate, making this the most northerly zone in Italy for the cultivation of the olive.
Variety: most of the olive trees are at least 100 years old, and the predominant variety is Casaliva, which is green at the harvest. Others found in small proportions include Grignano and Frantoio.

Picking: by hand from mid-November until February.
Method of Production: stone-crushed and cold pressed at the communal mill on Lake Garda. Filtered through cotton prior to bottling.
Acidity: 0.2–0.3 per cent.
General comments: the Allegrini family have 50 hectares of vineyard on the terraced hills of Valpolicella. Interspersed with the vines are olive trees, which here give a much softer oil than that found in Tuscany, although the acidity remains very low.

Here is everything a taster could wish to know about the pedigree of the oil. Samples taken on fresh crusty French bread would have been available at the wine/oil store.

Tastings in the Press
Sometimes tastings get into the Press. Usually there are panels of tasters, general chitchat about the oils and a score, with a picture of the label from the bottle. Below is an example of such write-ups. There is a good deal of information—date, area, price, merchant, country of origin and general impressions. (The price indicates it can only be Extra Virgin Olive Oil.) The initials indicate the tasters.

ITALY

Fattoria Selviapiana, Tuscany (1992)
£10.39 (50 cl) Winecellars tel: 0181-871-3979

From Chianti Rufina, a cooler area of Tuscany, this 'deep, murky green' (CM) oil wasn't giving too much away on the nose: hints of 'leaf and apple' spotted by CM. On the palate, the Frantoio olive brings that 'peppery finish' after 'earthy' (JR), 'heavy' (JH), 'great, fresh' (CM). 'Full of

24

character to use with beans or chicory salads' was Rose's tip.

Out of ten: 8

PACKAGING

However the oil is bottled, if the colour is a good luminous gold or green the bottle will be clear to show it off—a good colour makes any product attractive and saleable. Colours which are not so attractive can be found in green glass bottles which disguise the colour of the oil and give the product mood; they also help to preserve it by protecting it from the light.

Upmarket packaging freewheels into fancy bottles with corks, sealing wax, extra labels, attached cork and metal pourers, fancy lids and even gold foil covering the whole bottle. Murky-looking unfiltered oils in expensive bottles, olive oil and lemon juice blends, miniature bottles, olive oil with herbs steeping in it, gold labels, imitation straw and wooden boxes—the variety is endless. Whether the olive oil in these upmarket packages is any better than the plainly packaged oils off the supermarket shelf is debatable.

NUTRITIONAL VALUE

Olive oil is 100 per cent fat, has no protein, no carbohydrate, no sodium, no cholesterol, no minerals but a trace of vitamin E, which is fat soluble. One hundred grams of olive oil have a calorific value of 884. It is suitable for vegetarians and vegans as it is extracted from a fruit.

CHAPTER 2

The Chemistry of Olive Oil

Olive oil's constituents are organic chemicals. Chemistry is divided into two disciplines, inorganic and organic. It is unfortunate that in colloquial terms, organic has come to mean 'Naturally Made' with a very special place in consumers' vocabulary. Olive oil could be considered totally organic only if it was produced without pesticides and chemical fertilisers. Its composition in chemical terms is organic, but with a scientific meaning.

Organic chemistry is the study of all the chemicals of carbon. In its natural form, this will be familiar as charcoal, coal and diamonds. Olive oil is composed of long chains of carbon in combination with hydrogen and oxygen.

Long Chain Molecules

In organic chemistry, long chains of carbon, combined with hydrogen, form compounds known as paraffins and olefins. The carbon atom has four valencies or powers to bond with other atoms and can be represented as follows:

$$-\overset{\displaystyle |}{\underset{\displaystyle |}{C}}-$$

In simple terms, when each of the bonds is individually linked to another atom, the carbon atom is said to be saturated (a paraffin). If two of the bonds are linked

26

individually and the other two bonds (a double bond) are linked to just one atom, then the compound is said to be unsaturated and is depicted thus:

$$
\begin{array}{c}
\text{H} \\
| \\
\text{H} - \text{C} = \text{C} \ (\text{Olefins})
\end{array}
$$

In a long chain of carbon atoms, when the compound contains just one double bond, it is known as monounsaturated, but if there are more double bonds within the chain, it is polyunsaturated.

Long chain organic compounds may have acid groups attached to them and these can combine with alcohols to form stable compounds known as esters. Olive oil is composed of long chain acids linked to glycerine (an alcohol) which are esters known as triglycerides.

Long chain compounds containing from 16 to 24 carbon atoms in the chain are generally oily substances. When they have acid groups attached to them, they are called fatty acids.

Fatty Acids in Edible Fats
The fatty acid composition of all edible fats comprises three classes—saturated, monounsaturated and polyunsaturated. All these acids are combined as glycerine triglycerides. Listed below are the percentages of each of the three classes for a range of everyday oils (see Table 1). Please note, the figures in this table relate to the whole oil and include the glycerine content. In Table 2 (see p. 30) analysis is based upon total fatty acids with the glycerine ignored.

Olive oil is high in monounsaturated fatty acids, in particular oleic acid. At least half the triglycerides in olive oil are those of oleic acid which has a chain length consisting of 18 carbon atoms (C_{18}).

Table 1

	sat.	monounsat.	polyunsat.
Coconut	86.5	5.8	1.8
Rapeseed	5.6	62.4	27.7
Corn	12.7	24.4	58.7
Cottonseed	25.9	17.8	51.9
Grapeseed	9.6	16.1	69.9
Hazelnut	7.4	78.0	10.2
Olive	13.5	73.7	8.4
Palm	49.3	37.0	9.3
Peanut	16.9	46.0	32.0
Safflower	9.1	12.1	74.5
Sesame	14.2	39.7	41.7
Soyabean	14.4	23.3	57.9
Sunflower	10.3	19.5	65.7
Walnut	9.1	22.8	63.3

Ref: *Reader's Digest Complete Guide to Cooking*, Anne Willom

Unsaturated Oils

Chemically, unsaturated substances are always trying to become saturated, the saturated form being more stable than the unsaturated. Rancidity of oils takes place when the monounsaturated and polyunsaturated oils become saturated by oxidation and, in the process, are broken down to smaller, more stable molecules. The free fatty acids are much more likely to break down than those that are combined with glycerine as triglycerides. However, the presence of double bonds anywhere in a molecule gives inherent weakness and that is why, once a bottle of olive oil is opened, it should be used within a reasonable period of time.

It will be seen from Table 1 that olive oil contains saturated, monounsaturated and polyunsaturated fatty acids. The triglycerides formed by those acids are very large molecules and may be illustrated thus:

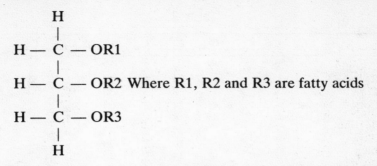

Within these compounds, the R figure may always be the same fatty acid or it may be three different fatty acids. Nature will probably have devised the triglyceride structures so as to minimise their rate of degradation. The more polyunsaturated fatty acids there are in edible oils, the more prone they are to rapid deterioration when exposed to the air.

Vitamin F
In the modern world, where more processed food is being consumed than ever before, the importance of using fresh edible oils cannot be overemphasised. The body needs polyunsaturates to use in vital body processes and at one time they were known as vitamins called Vitamin F Factors. When those polyunsaturates and monounsaturates are degraded, they become nutritionally worthless.

Fatty Acids in Edible Oils
Table 2 shows the percentage of individual fatty acids found in some commonly used oils.

Saturated Fats
It is generally accepted by nutritionists that consumption of excessive quantities of saturated fats is undesirable. This means that oils such as coconut and palm would not be such a good choice for food use as the other oils. The problem is

Table 2

	C_8	C_{10}	C_{12}	C_{14}	C_{16}	C_{18}	C_{18}''	$C_{18}2''$	C_{22}''
Coconut	9	8	46	17	9	2	7	2	–
Rapeseed	–	–	–	–	4	1	14	26	55
Corn	–	–	–	–	8	3	30	59	–
Cottonseed	–	–	–	3	24	2	23	48	–
Grapeseed	–	–	–	–	8	4	17	71	–
Hazelnut	–	–	–	–	5	3	82	10	–
Olive	–	–	–	–	10	3	78	9	–
Palm	–	–	–	2	43	5	40	10	–
Peanut*	–	–	–	–	8	3	56	26	–
Safflower	–	–	–	–	6	3	13	78	–
Sesame	–	–	–	–	9	6	45	40	–
Soyabean†	–	–	–	–	10	3	26	58	–
Sunflower	–	–	–	–	6	4	25	65	–
Walnut‡	–	–	–	–	6	3	18	63	–

* also contains 7% higher (i.e. $C_{24}+$)
† also contains 3% higher (i.e. $C_{24}+$)
‡ also contains 10% higher (i.e. $C_{24}+$)

Ref: *The Chemical Constituents of Natural Fats, T.P. Hilditch. Chapman Hall, 1957.*

that these oils are very stable and are therefore used widely by the food industry where it is important that processed foods have a long shelf life. There is an idea amongst consumers that all vegetable oils are better than animal fats. That is not so. It is the saturated fats which are not so desirable as the unsaturated for nutritional purposes.

Hydrogenated, Trans and Cis Fats
When a fat is 'hydrogenated', this means that it has been saturated by treating it with the gas hydrogen to break the double bonds and render it more stable for use in food processing and cooking. However, this process may produce trans fatty acids which are probably less desirable nutritionally than saturated fatty acids.

Safflower, sunflower, corn and soyabean oils are widely used in food and in home cooking because they contain relatively large amounts of polyunsaturated fatty acids.

Although there is no doubt about the potential role that polyunsaturated fatty acids play in the diet, there are certain problems surrounding their use. Modern agriculture has enabled varieties of plants to be selected to yield high levels of the desirable polyunsaturated fatty acids when they are harvested. However, some of these oils—for example, rapeseed, borage and blackcurrant—contain an undesirable fatty acid, known as erucic acid, within their composition. This has to be limited by law in oils for human consumption because of its adverse effects on the heart muscle. Whilst those oils might have a part to play in food processing, for those who are health conscious, any product containing rapeseed or borage should be avoided. Borage oil is also known as starflower oil.

Besides erucic acid, there are other undesirable fatty acids present in many vegetable oils, particularly hydrogenated ones. These are familiarly known as the trans isomers. Isomer is a chemical term relating to compounds of identical two-dimensional representation but which, when taken into the three-dimensional, become different. When two carbon atoms are joined together by a double bond, they cannot easily rotate as there are two nails, as it were, joining them together rather than just one. This is important in the three-dimensional view because a transposition of two groups attached to one of those carbon atoms will produce a compound of totally different three-dimensional configuration. In natural processes, particularly body metabolism, these differences can be crucial and can even result in a substance being poisonous to the body instead of being vital for its continuing existence.

As far as the nutritional use of fatty acids is concerned, a trans form is undesirable, but the cis form is essential. This

31

concept can be illustrated by the active constituent of olive oil, oleic acid, which in the cis form may be drawn as follows:

$$CH_3 - (CH_2)_7 - \overset{\displaystyle \overset{H}{|}}{C} = \overset{\displaystyle \overset{H}{|}}{C} - (CH_2)_7 - COOH$$

The trans form of the same molecule is known as elaidic acid:

$$\overset{\displaystyle CH_3\ (CH_2)7\ H}{\underset{\displaystyle H - C = C\ (CH_2)_7 - COOH}{|}}$$

There is now a strong body of opinion amongst doctors that trans fatty acids are harmful. Its high content of cis mono-unsaturate and the fact that it contains no trans fatty acids means that olive oil is one of the most desirable food oils we can include in our diet.

Human Body Fat and Olive Oil
It is interesting to compare the composition of olive oil with that of human body fat (see Table 3).

Table 3

	Female 54 years	Male 76 years	Male 61 years	Male 66 years	Olive Oil
C_{12}	0.1	0.6	–	0.9	–
C_{14}	2.7	5.9	2.6	3.9	–
C_{16}	24.0	25.0	24.7	25.7	10
C_{18}	8.4	5.8	7.7	5.2	3
C_{14}''	0.2	0.6	0.4	0.5	–
C_{16}''	5.0	6.7	7.3	7.6	–
C_{18}'' (oleic acid)	46.9	45.4	45.8	46.6	78
$C_{18}2''$	10.2	8.2	10.0	8.7	9
other unsat	2.5	1.8	1.5	0.9	–

Ref: Crayer, D. L. and Brown, J. B. J. *Biol Chem.*, 1943, 151, 427.

Several points are highlighted in this table. First, there is little or no difference between the male and female figures. Second, there is very little change with age; so it would be reasonable to suppose that these figures apply throughout life.

The most significant feature is that both the human body and olive oil have oleic acid as a major part of the fatty acid spectrum. Linoleic acid content is virtually the same too. Considering the importance of unsaturated fatty acids in life processes, perhaps the presence of this oil in what many doctors consider to be the healthiest diet in the Western world—the Mediterranean type of diet—has been overlooked too long and should now be considered alongside those other important factors in that diet, the major presence of Vitamins C and E, together with beta carotene. Olive oil must be the most compatible food oil for human nutritional purposes.

Adulteration and Analysis
As a highly prized (and rightly so) and expensive oil throughout the ages, adulteration by unscrupulous traders must always be considered a possibility. Chemical analysis can detect where adulteration has taken place and has been an important part of food and drug legislation for many years. Sometimes, adulteration can be very serious and lead to death, as in the notorious Spanish toxic oil syndrome epidemic of 1981: hundreds of people were killed and thousands left disabled. Using sophisticated methods of chemical analysis, adulteration can readily be detected.

Traders will look for cheaper oils with a very similar spectrum in the oleic and linoleic acid contents for their adulterants. But if you look at Table 2, you will see that all the oils have very distinctive compositions, and blending to try to mimic one oil would probably be more costly than using the pure materials. Oils which have been found as

33

popular adulterants of olive oil include corn oil, peanut oil (ground nut), sunflower and rapeseed oil. All these can be easily detected using straightforward analytical techniques.

BP Standards
Whilst olive oil generally available in the grocery trade is not labelled 'BP', it is almost certain that it has been analysed in accordance with the methods laid down in that important book of standards used by chemists and doctors, *The British Pharmacopoeia*. BP Standards include limit tests for cottonseed oils, nut oils and sesame oils. In addition, there are several tests designed to measure the rancidity of the oil. These include tests for iodine value, saponification value, peroxide value and acid value. Analysts will interpret the results of these tests and determine whether the oil is suitable for sale.

With modern technical laboratory equipment, it is possible to measure the concentrations of individual fatty acids present in edible oils. A machine called a gas liquid chromatograph can produce a computer trace which will be a fingerprint for practically any known oil. Any adulteration can be detected by comparing the spectrum obtained from the sample with that of a known standard.

CHAPTER 3

Olive Oil in the Diet

Anyone who shopped in an old-fashioned grocer's shop in the 1950s will have difficulty in remembering olive oil. It would have been in small glass bottles on the delicatessen shelf or counter. Sunflower and polyunsaturated margarine were nowhere on the scene but the huge blocks of butter, lard and hard margarine were still in evidence. Assistants spent hours cutting them and wrapping them in greaseproof paper.

There were no supermarkets as such but there was a legion of small grocers and corner shops with limited storage facilities, usually at the back of the premises. At that time it would have been almost impossible for olive oil to be sold widely. There was insufficient storage, little display area and most customers would not have known what to do with it as it was a luxury item. However, it was on sale everywhere in chemists' shops and could be dispensed by the pharmacists, without prescription, for putting in the ears or rubbing into the skin. Most medicine cupboards would have held a small bottle of it at that time, and some still do today.

Magazines and cookbooks did not feature the oil except as a rare ingredient, for we were still in the grip of the postwar excitement about the end of fat rationing. The influence was mainly on how to feed your family properly when there was not much money to go round; food was generally plain but nourishing and cooked by the housewife. The glamour side was French cooking, heavy with butter and cream.

As Britain is too cold for the cultivation of the olive it was natural that we should continue, as we have for centuries, to use fats from animals. It took cooks prepared to travel to make home cooks think about changing their ideas.

Elizabeth David travelled widely in Italy, France and other Mediterranean countries, seeking out traditional food and writing down the recipes that had been handed down from one generation to another. Her books appeared in paperback at an affordable price and opened up a whole new world for the home cook prepared to experiment and break away from traditional British food.

The Sixties saw shortages as a distant memory and far more varieties of food appeared in the shops which were suitable for European-type cooking. The Common Market, by expanding, made more foods available for export to Britain. Better forms of transport, new roads and easier communication with overseas producers made getting foods to the consumer much easier. One of those foods was olive oil but the place to buy it was the delicatessen, not the grocer or the supermarket. It was still very much a luxury item.

FOOD AND HEALTH

By the end of the 1970s health was becoming an important issue. Although lambasted by the media, new ideas about a healthier style of eating took hold. Junk food, however, which was becoming really big business, is noted for its aggressive marketing. No opportunity was lost to discredit the idea of healthy eating. The mere fact that olive oil for cooking is an expanding market shows that the common sense of the consumer is prevailing, whatever the pressure from the media, because health is now a big issue in the supermarket. Magazines have given it lip-service to an extent but on TV, the mainstay of junk food advertising, there has been little if anything positive about making the diet healthier. There seems to be no happy medium in the matter.

People are more adventurous with their food in Britain because they can now travel easily to all parts of the world and are exposed to many different cultures, enjoying a wide variety of foods. Pizza and hamburger takeaways have taken over largely from fish and chip shops which were everywhere in the 1950s and '60s. They went into a steep decline when the price of fish rose due to overfishing and quotas, and nosedived when oven-ready frozen fish and chips became available. The 1976 drought caused a severe shortage of potatoes and the price rocketed. For many fish and chip shops this was the straw that broke the camel's back.

Chinese, Indian, Asian and Italian restaurants and take-aways have also replaced some of the fish and chip shops. The popularity of Italian food, especially pasta, is stagger-ing and this is a factor that has helped to establish the olive oil market in the UK. Salads are also very popular because they don't require cooking and are available, ready pre-pared, in supermarkets. With the popularity of salad cream on the wane, olive oil and similar-based vinaigrettes are an easily made dressing and merely have to be shaken up in a bottle. The raw egg scare added somewhat to the loss of popularity in mayonnaise for a while and this, too, helped to make olive oil or other oil-based vinaigrettes popular. Rows of them are now to be found in every supermarket.

Despite the increasing awareness of healthy eating among a minority of the population, since the mid-1980s the general trend has been for the worse. Ready meals and processed food have taken over the market and cooking at home is on the wane. With a microwave oven all that is required is to unwrap a pack from the freezer and give the contents a quick warm-up. Fast food shops have sprung up everywhere and some young people have begun to live totally on processed food. Cooking skills are no longer passed from mother to daughter—there are few to pass on. Although seasonal foods are now available all year round and shortages rarely occur, the national diet is probably the worst it has been this century.

Health Problems and Diet

As medical research progressed, it became clear that the high saturated fat, cholesterol-rich, high sugar and salt, low fibre, too few fresh fruit and vegetables (or none at all) kind of diet most people were (and still are) having, was leading to avoidable health problems such as heart disease. With an extremely high rate of this health nasty—much higher than in other Western countries—alarm bells began to ring and are still ringing.

The Mediterranean diet has now become a popular concept. Public opinion now links good health and low incidence of heart disease squarely on this way of eating. It is even more popular because smoking and drinking (alcohol) and white bread are not big issues in places like Italy. In Mediterranean areas they are a way of life.

The Mediterranean diet is one which has small amounts of red meat, chicken being the main source of meat protein, along with plenty of fish, pulses and, near the coast, shellfish. It has plenty of fresh fruit and vegetables, usually in the form of salad. Pasta and rice are the main carbohydrate foods, along with good bread. The main fat in the diet is provided by olive oil at the expense of butter and margarine.

It would be naive to suppose that it is only the use of olive oil which makes the diet a healthy one, but this is emerging as a popular myth, not helped by the UK media who have a tendency to see everything as black and white with seemingly little attention to truth or detail. In media-speak a new highly saturated spread would be seen as a 'killer fat' and a monounsaturated oil as a 'heart saver'. TV and radio broadcasting, with a few exceptions, have a tradition of making a joke out of food, cooking and health. Most cookery programmes are still trotting out 1950s cholesterol celebration recipes (known as 'heart attack cookery') and have not moved with the times. Health is not yet an important TV issue except as a novelty, so the situation is rather stagnant. Really the mainstream food programmes are to cooking what the many violent programmes are to crime: the policy seems to be not to change.

Margarine
At the turn of the century a kind of margarine was already available in Britain. It was cheaper than butter, kept better and looked very similar. It was called 'butterine' and was unpopular among country folk who were used to using lard from their own pig, either spread with mustard or sprinkled with fresh rosemary. Children would have it with a 'scraping of black treacle or sprinkling of brown sugar'. The spread was used on thickly sliced bread and was an important part of a rather restricted diet.

Highly saturated block margarines followed and persist to this day. However, soft spreads have more appeal as they are not only easier to spread but much easier to use in baking. Anyone who has literally beaten hard margarine and sugar to a light cream, by hand, will have had an aching arm to prove it!

Margarine now provides another way into the UK diet for olive oil. It began in London in 1991 when a new kind of margarine was launched. The first olive oil margarine-like spread, named Olivio and developed by Van den Berghs, is a reduced fat spread (60 per cent fat) positioned between margarine (80 per cent fat) and low fat spread (40 per cent fat). Its advantage is that it can be used in cooking, which low fat spreads cannot. Packed in an attractive tub in 250g and 500g sizes, it is priced to be cheaper than butter. By 1994 it was in every supermarket with a market share and an amazing growth rate of +90 per cent per year. Its positioning is based on 'the goodness and purity of olive oil' and it was put on the market when Van den Berghs recognised that UK consumers were becoming increasingly aware of the 'benefits of the oil, the Mediterranean diet and the monounsaturates, in health terms'.

Like most successful products it was copied. Several supermarket chains launched their own copycat products, so for olive oil spread users there is now a choice of brands.

Margarine, meanwhile, is an 'out' word due to EC directives, and products we all accept as margarine now have to be called 'spreads'. (Too bad the last 50 years of cookbooks are now wrong on this subject.) The new olive oil spreads are soft, yellow and on the bland side. The striving to equal the attractive taste of butter seems to have disappeared. Olive oil spread, it appears, is here to stay. This is good news for our health and for olive oil!

CHAPTER 4

Health

From the viewpoint that the lower incidence of heart attacks in Mediterranean countries coincides with consumption of olive oil, there has been some move among medical researchers towards the idea that the structure of the whole diet is involved, not just the oil. The Mediterranean diet is now being closely studied.

It should be borne in mind, however, that diet is only one piece of the jigsaw and that there are other factors which are different from life in Britain—some better, some worse.

Climate

There is no doubt that life in countries such as Italy, Greece or France is quite different from that of the UK. Starting with climate, we have a higher rainfall, colder winters and less sunshine. They endure more heat in their summers. What they accept as a normal summer, we find sweltering and uncomfortable when it happens here. Their homes are equipped for heat, with shutters and cool ceramic-tiled floors. We have large windows by choice and fitted carpets. Because the heat of the day is at its greatest between noon and four o'clock, they have *siesta*. This divides the working day into two distinct parts: early morning until noon and four until seven, with a rest or sleep in between. In the UK there is no such time for relaxation in the day, apart from the lunch hour 'break' when it is time for most people to do their shopping.

Fuel bills for heating in the colder British Isles are a

major household expense in the winter, especially for the elderly. Central heating is costly to run and open fires are rare because of smokeless zones. In Mediterranean countries, logs on an open hearth are the common form of winter heating and fuel is cheap.

Physical Fitness

Most people in the UK don't take enough in the way of exercise. A small proportion exercise too much. There is a network of sport and fitness centres, classes and playing fields for ball sports. Games and sports at school have declined as essential parts of the curriculum. Going out for a walk has become dangerous and frightening due to the levels of crime, such as mugging, so this too has declined. A great many cars pollute the atmosphere in the towns and cities and walking is not the pleasure it was. Some areas are overrun with tourists making the local population feel their space has been invaded.

In some Mediterranean areas, people still walk a good deal. In Italy and France, where the café society prevails, most people go for a walk in the early evening. In Greece the ratio of cars to people is high and pollution is frightening in Athens, where most of the population live. Some days, when there is no breeze, traffic is banned altogether due to the dangerous level of exhaust fumes that cannot escape. In Mediterranean countries there are still peasants who work the land and do a good deal of physically hard work, although since the EC was formed, there has been more mechanisation to make it easier. All around the Mediterranean coast, the fishing industry thrives using small boats and nets; the British fishing industry has shrunk as the waters around the British Isles have been fished out by enormous nets. Fishermen are now a rarity. Farms are highly mechanised except where there are large flocks of sheep.

Work and Wages

Only a small proportion of the British population does hard physical work for a living. Working age women are largely overworked if they have a full-time job and also children to rear. The one-parent family is common and this kind of life is harder than one where there are two parents who can bring in a wage. With family life having largely disintegrated, life in the UK is more insecure and difficult.

In the Mediterranean countries, family ties are stronger. Baby-sitters are almost unheard of as there is always someone from the family willing to take responsibility for young and old as well. Families still sit down to meals together in cafés, tavernas and brasseries and, more important, at home. Children are welcome everywhere in places to eat. In the UK this is not so and we do not have a great tradition for it. Family mealtimes seem to have died out with the family.

Mentality

Whether climate plays a part in the mentality of people is difficult to say but certainly, in sunnier climates than ours, people do seem happier and more cheerful. The British are almost obsessed by the weather which can be very wet, depressing and changeable. The weather forecasters, of whom there seem to be many, often get it wrong. It is as if our weather is unreliable!

We have a reputation for 'reserve'. That means a kind of exterior coldness of manner and unwillingness to express emotion. Our Mediterranean counterparts have no such problem and are given to openly showing emotion (sometimes too much), and bold responses to emotional situations. They are especially good at grieving, which we don't seem to be.

43

Age

People in Mediterranean countries age more quickly in appearance than people in the UK. This is partly due to the ravages of the sun and wind. The moister climate in Britain helps to keep skin from drying too much and winter weather keeps us indoors. When it comes to longevity, however, the Mediterranean countries win. People who die aged over one hundred are not uncommon and the average age at which people die in Mediterranean countries is rather higher than in the UK; so longevity has become associated with the Mediterranean diet and olive oil.

Diet

The diet in the UK has changed considerably this century. By contrast, in Mediterranean countries it has not changed for centuries and it differs strikingly from the UK diet:

Bread

Bread is an important staple as potatoes are not eaten a great deal. Rice and pasta are the other two high carbohydrate foods. Small bakers are everywhere, baking seven days a week, two or three times a day. Bread is made from unbleached white flour or high gluten to make a crust. Brown bread is not eaten a great deal and only a minority buy it. Everybody in Mediterranean countries seems to have access to really good bread—a simple pleasure of everyday life largely missing in the UK.

Meat and Fish

Freshly slaughtered meat and freshly caught fish and shell-fish have to be eaten quickly because of the climate. Consequently they don't travel far. Locally produced meat from small farms and fish from the local fisherman are plentiful, without the wholesaler and shop between the farmer and fisherman. All around the coast, fish is bought on the quay as the little boats come in. Most people don't have large freezers as we do in the UK and eat fresh, not frozen food. Lamb and pork are the main types of meat; beef and horse are also available. Chicken from the small farms is the main source of meat protein.

Vegetables and Fruit

Again, due to the climate, fruit and vegetables don't stay fresh for long and are not made to travel too far. The range of vegetables does not vary much from one country to the next. In the hottest areas, the vegetable and fruit skins are rather tough. Root vegetables find it hard to put down their roots into the dry soil and vegetables like carrots can be rather coarse and fibrous. Potatoes are more difficult to grow than in the colder climate of more northerly countries. Peppers, aubergines, tomatoes, asparagus, many kinds of lettuce, spinach, cucumber, celery and onions grow easily and quickly and these form the basis of the vegetables eaten. Apart from spinach, aubergines and asparagus, they are all raw salad vegetables. Salad is eaten a great deal as a side dish or *hors d'oeuvre*. It is usually dressed with an olive oil vinaigrette, with the remains of the dressing mopped up with bread so as not to waste the oil. There is not the tradition of slow oven roasting and cooking that we have in the UK. Kebabs, quickly (shallow) fried food, or spit roasted meat and fish, bread and salad seem to be the centuries-old fare that everyone enjoys. There is not a great deal of variety, the appeal of the food resting on its colour and freshness.

In the hottest areas, a large platter of plain fresh fruit chunks with ice cubes serves as a pudding. Melon, apples, pears and grapes, sometimes with pineapple, or large slices of watermelon and melon, suffice. Our tradition of complicated fat-rich puddings served with cream or custard does not exist in Mediterranean countries. Ice cream seems to be their only indulgence. In Italy large fruit tarts as well as ice cream concoctions are popular. The farther north the pudding, the more likely it is to be from the patisserie.

The Fat of the Land

Butter is one UK fat of the land because we have a large dairy industry; so are cheese and cream, and to an extent full fat milk, creamy yoghurt and ice cream, lard and suet. In Mediterranean countries olive oil is the fat of the land. Although cheese is eaten there, it is usually served as an *hors d'oeuvre*, on salad, in a sauce or as a topping. However it is served it does not appear in large amounts. Ewes' and goats' milk are used for cheese as not all the pasture is suitable for herds of cows.

Eggs are used in the UK as a daily source of protein. They are also a cheap source of cholesterol! Eggs are not used so much in Mediterranean cooking. Apart from the French and Spanish omelette, they probably turn up more as a garnish than part of a main meal.

Bread is traditionally eaten without butter, as olive oil is put on the table and drizzled on bread or toast in preference. Since meat is not eaten in large quantities, the amount of animal fat in the diet is much smaller than in the UK.

Smoking

Whilst there are some measures in the UK to combat smoking, such as bans on advertising on TV, in the Mediterranean countries there seems to be no restraint. In the UK it is illegal to show a picture or photos of people smoking; all over the Mediterranean countries are hoardings of glamorous men and women puffing away. Generally there does not seem to be much concern for the health risks of smoking. Smoking in public is socially acceptable and cigarettes are cheap. As it is known to lead to respiratory complaints, high cholesterol, emphysema, poor circulation in feet and hands, and restricted capillary blood flow, this does indicate a blatant disregard for health. In spite of this attitude, they are healthier than we are.

Alcohol
In Mediterranean countries alcohol is much cheaper than in the UK where it is highly taxed. The vine flourishes where the olive does and regular drinking of wine is part of the lifestyle. In moderation it is said to lower cholesterol.

Fibre
Fruit, vegetables and pulses are the main source of dietary fibre. Wheat bran is conspicuous by its absence in the Mediterranean diet.

Water
A good deal of plain spring water is drunk throughout the day in the Mediterranean countries. Water is always put on the table at mealtimes, and during excessively hot spells extra water is drunk and a good deal is lost in perspiration. We do not drink anything like the same amount of plain water in the UK, mainly because we don't have hot weather. The health benefits of the water habit should not be overlooked. In hot weather it is drunk instead of coffee and there are often water fountains in public places or bottled water on sale.

Changes
All these are really generalities and there are exceptions. With the fast food industry taking more of a hold in Mediterranean countries, tourism sets up a new kind of food demand, and with processed food imports the Mediterranean diet is becoming less healthy. Experts were

reading for the diet not to change years ago. Since then, with the gradual swing to a less healthy diet, the heart attack and illness rate has begun to rise.

FATS AS NUTRIENTS

We all need some fat in our diet, but it should be some of each kind, saturates, polyunsaturates and monounsaturates. The unsaturated fatty acid oleic acid is present in all fats to an extent but found in high concentration in olive oil. We need fat to enable us to eat our food, to keep us warm and to carry vitamins A, D, E and K around the body. These four are fat soluble, that is they dissolve in fat rather than water. Vitamin D is important for healthy bones, heart, nerves, skin, teeth and thyroid glands; vitamin A is for healthy bones, hair, eyes, skin and teeth; vitamin E is for healthy blood vessels, heart, lungs, nerves and skin and vitamin K for healthy blood and liver.

We also need fats for a very important reason: they contain essential fatty acids. They belong to the vitamin F family and are linoleic, linolenic, gamma-linolenic and arachidonic acids. They are known as EFAs and the last two can be made by the body by converting linolenic acid to gamma-linolenic acid and then to arachidonic acid. Every living cell in our bodies requires them. The liver also needs fats for a special reason.

The liver produces bile continuously, storing it in the gall bladder. Bile helps with the work of digesting carbohydrate and protein and the absorption of the fat soluble vitamins A, D, E and K. It also plays a part in signalling the start of the digestive process, causing saliva and gastric juices to flow, and stimulates the production of a hormone required for digestion. Bile contains bile salts which help in the digestion of fats by making them into minute droplets.

48

As we saw in Chapter 1, the liver also uses fat to manufacture cholesterol which, in reasonable amounts, is essential to health.

FAT LEVELS

In the UK the average person is eating too much in the way of fat. Every year there are 160 deaths from heart disease for every 100,000 people. Until the fat intake is reduced the figures will not change. In Mediterranean countries the death rate is far lower. Polyunsaturated fat has enjoyed a reputation second to none for over twenty years as the healthiest of fats; now it is gradually being toppled as olive oil benefits are medically proven in trials.

Daily Intake of Fats

As we need some of each of polyunsaturated, saturated and monounsaturated fat daily, olive oil will take care of the latter. About a tablespoon of oil a day would seem to be a sensible amount. Saturated fat in meat, butter, cheese and cream, polyunsaturated fat from sunflower or safflower oil or polyunsaturated margarines will easily make up the other two.

Obviously, there is no point in going 100 per cent over to olive oil as we need a variety of fats. However, there is one weak spot in the UK diet which allows a good deal of saturated fat—chips. Oils for cooking chips by the deep fry method may be highly saturated. This explodes the myth that if an oil is clear it is unsaturated. The same applies to 'soft' margarines high in polyunsaturates. Hydrogenated fat used in their manufacture as a means of preventing rancidity falls into the saturated class.

Olive oil, although high in monounsaturates, also contains 15 per cent saturated fat and 12 per cent polyunsaturated fat. Coconut and palm oils which are both prized for commercially produced biscuits, deep frozen foods, pastry and cakes, are highly saturated fats.

HEALTH REPORT

When the (British) National Committee on Nutrition Education finally completed its report in 1983, it was suppressed because its findings were so critical about the quality of manufactured and processed food consumption in the UK. It also contained suggestions linking the general health of the nation to the poor food we eat. Heart attacks, strokes, obesity, diabetes, gout, constipation, diverticulitis and so on were bandied about in the press but without much sincerity. A major shift in eating habits means a major crisis on the agricultural front and in the massive junk food industry. More food mountains and higher unemployment naturally follow; so too could a population with better health and lower NHS costs.

Since the NACNE report was published, other studies such as the COMA report have followed in much the same vein. Still nothing much has been done about the situation and, if anything, things seem to have got worse regarding the health quality of the national diet. At the same time, the money to be made from inferior and processed food (junk food) has increased. There are now many more opportunities to eat an unhealthy diet. Meanwhile the queues for the surgery grow longer and the NHS is tottering under the weight of bureaucracy, having seemingly turned itself into an organisation for its employees rather than the sick.

CHANGING TIMES IN BRITAIN

Although, in the past few centuries, poor housing, lack of sanitation, poor water supplies, poverty and inadequate diet have been the main causes of illness and disease, the improvement in all but the last factor has had a tremendously positive effect on the population. People are living much longer and the potential burden of the elderly is already weighing down on the working population.

Instead of not eating enough, we are now eating too much. The population is unhealthy but in a different way from when poverty was the main factor. We have disease and illness from overeating some foods and not eating enough of others. This occurs against a background of a time of plenty. Food shops are everywhere, stacked high with thousands of foods. Some of our farmland is subsidised by the government to lie fallow ('setaside'). We don't need any more food, we already have too much.

Education
Although people in Britain ate a much better diet for their health in World War II due to shortages and rationing, no lesson seems to have been learnt from this triumph in a time of great adversity. Education regarding a better diet has failed time after time. Doctors seem to know as little about what to eat to keep healthy as their patients do.

This is depressing; as far back as far as several centuries BC the ancient Greeks understood very well what a good healthy diet would do for the human body. Their sculptures of athletes bear witness to perfection of the human body. This cannot be achieved by fatty takeaways, fizzy drinks, salty snacks and chocolate bars.

However, there are one or two glimmers of light. Olive oil is now being advertised. This may only be to boost the fortunes of the producers and retailers but, probably unbeknown to them, they are contributing to the improved health of the nation. Olive oil is becoming fashionable and sales are going up at the rate of 20 per cent annually. Olive

51

oil margarines, as we saw in Chapter 3, are creeping ւ,ɔ on
the polyunsaturated market and are being advertised.

MEDITERRANEAN/UK DIET

It is not difficult to follow the good principles of a Mediterranean diet in the UK, or to devise an even healthier one.
Part of that diet should be olive oil, but not to excess.

Basically the following are wrong with the British diet:
too much fat of the wrong kind, too much salt and sugar,
too little fibre, fresh fruit and vegetables.

Anyone now confused about what a healthy diet might
be, can study the following table which can be used, not as
a strict regime but merely as a guide.

BASIC DIET FOR HEALTH

Suggested Amounts of Food for One Adult for One Week

HIGH VITAMIN/MINERAL FOODS

Vegetables	allow at least one portion of leafy greens per day
	3 oz (75 g) frozen vegetables
	2 lb (1.5 kg) potatoes (fresh)
	2½ lb (1.25 kg) fresh green and other vegetables
Fruit	over 2 lb (1 kg) fresh fruit
	3 oz (75 g) dried fruit and nuts
	2 oz (50 g) canned fruit without sugar
HIGH FAT/OIL FOODS	7 fl oz (225 ml) olive oil
	3 oz (75 g) polyunsaturated margarine (now called 'spread')
	2 oz (50 g) butter (saturated fat)
	2 fl oz (50 ml) oil high in polyunsaturates such as sunflower, safflower, corn, soya.

	4 oz (110 g) cheese, preferably low fat
Alcohol	not more than 3 glasses wine daily (3 bottles per week)
Beverages	about 2½ oz (65 g) tea, coffee, cocoa, etc.
Other foods	9 oz (250 g)

HIGH SUGAR FOODS

Sugar	not more than 5 oz (150 g)
Jam/sweet spreads	4 oz (110 g)
Biscuits	4 oz (110 g), or 1 per day
Cakes/buns, pastries	under 3 oz (75 g), or about 2 items per week

HIGH CARBOHYDRATE FOODS

Pulses	1½ (40 g) dried beans, split peas, lentils etc.
Rice/wholewheat	1 lb (450 g), or 2 portions of rice
Pasta/noodles	and 3 portions of pasta
Flour	about 6 oz of wholewheat
Bread	1¼ lb (550 g) wholewheat/granary high fibre
	12 oz (350 g) white
	4 oz (110 g) of other breads
Breakfast cereals	8 oz (225 g), or about 5 portions

HIGH PROTEIN FOODS

Meat lean only from about 2 lb (1 kg) weight; bone, gristle and fat to be discarded	4½ oz (125 g) beef/veal/lamb
	1½ oz liver
	1½ sausages (low fat)
	2½ oz lamb
	4 oz (110 g) bacon/ham/pork
	12 oz (330 g) poultry
	4½ oz (125 g) other meat products
Fish	1 lb (450 g) mixed fresh and canned fish, shellfish

Milk	about 2 pints (1 litre) skimmed milk
	2 small yoghurts (plain)
Eggs	4

Cookery Advice

Wherever possible, meat should be trimmed of excess fat before cooking. Grill rather than fry and avoid deep fat frying as a method of cooking.

Preference should be given to fresh fruit and vegetables rather than canned, frozen or processed varieties.

Cook jacket potatoes and eat the skin as well as the flesh. Boil new potatoes in their skins.

Avoid salt in cooking and at table if possible.

Make your own pasta at home with wholewheat flour.

Use brown rice in preference to white.

Use the stir/cook method for vegetables at least three times per week.

Eat a raw salad at least five times a week.

Eat one good portion of a leafy green vegetable every day.

Eat bread three times a day to use up the bread allowance and if possible make your own or buy from the old-fashioned kind of small bakery. Eat it mostly without butter/margarine.

Have three portions of fresh fruit daily and five portions of fresh vegetables, including a green leafy one.

Avoid junk food, salty snacks, fizzy drinks.

Add fresh fruit to yoghurt to make flavoured yoghurt.

ALLERGY

A note here about this distressing medical condition which often requires a strict exclusion and avoidance of preparations. Those allergic to the seed and bean oils, such as sunflower, safflower, sesame, grape, soya, or to grain and nut oils such as peanut, palm, walnut, hazelnut and maize, often find olive oil a godsend as it is a fruit oil. It is also useful for the milk allergic who cannot eat butter or margarines which contain whey. Very few people are allergic to olive oil but it is a recognised allergen. It is more likely to occur among populations where olive oil is used as a staple and so is extremely rare in the UK where wheat, milk and eggs are thought to be the three major allergens.

Exclusions

The olive oil allergic needs to follow a diet which excludes the oil itself, and any food or products which may contain the oil—salad dressing, mayonnaise, fried food, commercially prepared/convenience foods; shampoos, soaps, conditioners, cosmetic creams, bath oils, tanning oils, cosmetics. As it is expensive, olive oil is not used as much commercially as other oils, but, it is still used in industry and crops up in the most unlikely items. Best advice is for the olive oil allergic to cross olive oil off the shopping list and turn to DIY for soaps, shampoo, cosmetics and toiletries.

*   *   *

You will have seen in this chapter how different the diet and lifestyle are in Mediterranean countries compared with the UK. There are pluses and minuses in each country but overall the Mediterranean countries seem to have a situation which makes them enjoy health. It is now part of myth and folklore that healthier heart and circulation and longevity are due to olive oil and science is backing it up. It remains to be seen if the same beneficial effects will be evident in the UK now that olive oil is taking a hold in the market.

CHAPTER 5

Tastes, Aromas, and Colours

As the twenty-first century approaches, so the range and availability of olive oil to the consumer grows. What was once a rarity in the UK is now in every supermarket. Olive oil plain, olive oil flavoured, olive oil blended with other oils; ranks of bottles rubbing shoulders with the rest of the market—sunflower, safflower, groundnut, soya, grapeseed, vegetable, sesame, walnut, hazelnut; everyday culinary oils and specialist oils. They are oils for frying, baking, marinades and salad dressings and are now a basic grocery item.

Flavoured Oils
Olive oil for culinary use comes in a wide variety of flavours for use with or in food, as a condiment, or a medicine. For cosmetics and other products the flavour does not matter. Flavours can be introduced to the oil by mixing or steeping herbs in it.

Flavoured oils are made by steeping fresh herbs in the oil. Herb flavours such as tarragon, basil, garlic, mint, fennel, marjoram, thyme, rosemary and savory can be imparted to the oil quite easily. Half fill a jar with the fresh herb, fill with olive oil, cover and leave to steep in a dark place for one to two weeks. If using garlic, four or five cloves cut in halves will flavour a small bottle of oil.

Harvests
As with all oil-rich crops, there are good, bad and indifferent harvests and excellent, good, poor, indifferent and

bad quality oils as a result. With many varieties of olives grown all over the world where the climate is suitable, on varied soils, with harvests ready at different times of the year and a variety of coloured fruit, it is obvious there will be a diverse range of quality, colour, aroma, flavour and slight difference in the levels of acidity of the oil produced.

Off Flavours

At the bottom end of the market are unpleasant 'off flavour' olive oils with six main taste/aroma categories of failure to please—*cucumber*, *flat* or *smooth*, *harsh*, *rancid* and *old*.

Oil which has stood too long is said to taste of *cucumber* or just taste *old*. *Rancid* is self-explanatory. It is a distasteful flavour which befalls all fats and oils which have had too much contact with the air. Alas, nothing can correct this flavour. Olive oil which produces an astringent feel in the mouth is said to be *harsh*, and when an olive oil has a flavour and aroma so weak as to be characterless it is described as *flat* or *smooth*. Some olive oils feel too greasy in the mouth and would be classed as *fatty*.

Bad Flavours

Common sense will tell you that bad practices will produce bad oils and the following are the result of husbandry and milling that have gone badly wrong, or just poor harvests. Olives preserved in a saline solution have a *brine* flavour. Poor washing of olives with earth or mud on them are described as *earthy* as the dirt supersedes the olive. New esparto mats for pressing usually make the oil taste more of the mats than the olives. This flavour is called *esparto*. Dirty pressing mats containing previous pressing residue (fermented) have a *pressing mat* flavour. Olives allowed to ferment because of poor storage can taste *fusty*. Mineral oils, petrol and grease from machinery will make olives smell *greasy*. *Green leaves* is a flavour not so much from the olives but from leaves and twigs that have not been removed before crushing. Excessively green olives will also produce this flavour.

Nutty Flavours
The nutty flavours come with sweet olive oils. One has been compared to fresh or dried *almonds*. The latter is easily confused with rancidity and is therefore not thought to make a good oil. *Hazelnut* and *walnut* are two distinct, self-explanatory flavours/aromas. Just plain *nutty* describes a general flavour much as you would find in a good wholewheat slice of bread.

EC-Approved Olive Oil Speak
The EC-approved terms are just a part of all those already discussed. Bureaucrats have their own way of controlling everything. Here is olive oil taste/aroma description reduced to EC speak, at a distance from the olive tree, olive oil, the producers and the consumers.

> Astringent, bitter, fruity, ripely fruity, sweet, apple, grass, hay, almond, cucumber, flat or smooth, harsh, old, rancid, brine, earthy, esparto, greasy, green leaves, grubby, heated or burnt, metallic, muddy sediment, mustiness-humidity, pomace, pressing mat, rough, soapy, vegetable water, winey-vinegary.

(It is comforting to think that anyone can go to an olive oil shop or department and come away with just the oil to suit them, without knowing any of this.)

Subjectivity
While it is difficult to be exact when describing aromas and flavours of olive oil, fanciful alternatives are often used for

promotion, or through national fervour and enthusiasm. Bear in mind we are dealing with an oil whose taste and aroma may only *hint* at a particular food/experience. Thus the descriptive language for olive oil may be at a slight distance from correctness, sheltering under the umbrella of 'subjectivity'.

Basically, when tasting, the *style* of an oil must be considered. This is a first impression and, unlike wine, nothing to do with colour. *Green* or *bitter* describes the taste of oil from green olives and those just turning colour. If it is an intense taste it will probably be unpleasant, otherwise it is typical of olive oil.

An instant impact from an oil when tasted is referred to as *bite*. Not all olive oils have this characteristic. Others with a strong aroma or flavour are said to have *depth*, or to be *strong*. Those with a weaker aroma and flavour come into the *light* or *mild* category.

A slightly sweet taste is present in some olive oils. These are actually called *sweet* or sometimes *ripely fruity*. Ripe fruit will sometimes produce this type of oil which has a somewhat weak aroma. The word *smooth* is largely a derogatory term and describes oils without a great deal of character regarding aroma and taste. You have already encountered it linked with an even more derogatory term, *flat*, earlier in this chapter. However, many tasters would say this was too harsh a judgement.

Pungent, *piccante*, *fruity*, *astringent* and *aromatic* are all forceful adjectives and apply to the more robust kinds of olive oil. *Pungent* means a strong-flavoured oil with a touch of bitterness—enough to make it interesting rather than unpleasant. (A parallel would be the bitter taste of a bitter lemon drink.) An oil which gives the taster a hot, spicy, peppery sensation at the back of the throat is described by the word *piccante*. *Astringent* is used to describe a sensation of many flavours at once, such as when tannins are present in the mouth. (Tea has a good tannin content.)

Distinct from these robust flavours are the (seemingly) fruit-flavoured olive oils. There are nine of these—*apple*, *banana*, *lemon peel*, *ripe melon*, *orange peel*, *passion fruit*, *cooked*, *fresh pears*, *tomato skins* or *fresh tomato juice*.

Against these there are only four (seemingly) vegetable flavours. They are *avocado*, *artichokes*, *asparagus*, and *mushrooms*.

Peasant describes a peasant/rustic kind of flavour which is not entirely complimentary. *Freshly mown grass* or *hay* (dried grass) are two suggestive flavours. An oil that is reminiscent of a bouquet of flowers is classed as *floral* or *flowery*. *Leafy* is more on the herbaceous side and can be influenced by its green colour.

Harmony and Balance

So much for flavour and aroma. Now is the time to consider the harmony and balance of an olive oil taste, which can usually be described by one of the following: aggressive, delicate, fragrant, harmonious, mellow, rich, rounded or rustic.

Olive oil needs to have a strong punchy flavour to win the title *aggressive*. An assault on the taste buds which makes the taster feel he has had a confrontation with the oil will fall into this quick impression category.

Mellow oils, *soft* and *sweet* oils and *delicate* oils which are both aromatic and light appear gentler flavoured and lightly scented. By contrast, oils with a full rounded flavour are classed as *rich*. *Rustic* denotes a robust, hearty flavour and aroma and *rounded* is used to describe what is considered a well balanced oil. *Fragrant* is a complex aromatic with a hint of flower scent. This is a general scent and not one particular flower. *Harmonious*, which sounds rather Chinese in concept, applies to oils which have good ratios of all aroma and taste factors.

Variety

What, you might ask, gives rise to this staggering array of aromas and flavours! Quality, variety of olive, soil, climate, cultivation, harvesting, pressing, sometimes blending, and the age of an oil all have a part to play. Note that colour does not, although it can play a subjective part when the oil is tasted, so much so that, as we saw in Chapter 1, it has sometimes to be hidden from the taster in a coloured glass.

COLOURS OF OLIVE OIL

Although colour is not always an indicator of taste, aroma or quality or even of the colour of the olives from which it has been produced, it is worth a mention.

Mrs Beeton's *Training Cookbook* (1923 New Edition, 3000 Practical Recipes) gave this advice on colour:

> *Tests for Foods*
> Olive oil is so valuable an item in the kitchen that it is well to know which is the best kind. A deep brownish-yellow or dark green oil should be avoided. The very best quality is a light green, while oil that is almost colourless or that shading to a golden yellow, may be used safely.

Imagine a colour range from pale lemony gold, through mid golden greens to a deep yellow green. Some green oils are not particularly pleasant on the eye—acid green, depressing green, poison green; a mixture of chrome yellow and Prussian blue would give a range of these on the artist's palette. More typical would be a mixture of lemon yellow and black with tints and shades from light to dark.

CHAPTER 6

Kitchen and Cupboard

There are olive oils for salads, frying, marinades, baking and cosmetics. Do not be too influenced by the colour of the oil when you are buying. The important factor is the taste. If you can buy at a specialist shop where you are able to taste and be given advice, don't miss the opportunity. If you are buying without tasting, smaller sizes of bottle are for you; there is no real answer to the expensive mistake.

Regrettably, you will have to take pot luck as labels are misleading. 'A light salad oil' can mean an oil from a third refined (hot) pressing. The Extra Virgin or Virgin (both unrefined) labels are there to help you and the price will also be an indicator of quality. If you are in a position to buy three quite different oils, then do so; they will give you the variety you need to become an enthusiastic user.

Storage
Having chosen your olive oil, whether for culinary or cosmetic use, do store it in a cool dark place to stop it going rancid. Now that the larder has largely disappeared, the fridge has taken over as a mini-larder. Olive oil stored in the fridge is apt to turn semi-solid and is best not used straight from the fridge. It will return to its normal consistency at room temperature, so should be taken out of the fridge well before it is required. You can see how the cool, dark place is more convenient than the fridge. Bear in mind, time and light are the two things which will spoil olive oil.

Bulk Buying

If you are buying a large amount—say enough to last a year—decant into small bottles and store them in the dark. Really, from a practical point of view it is better to buy smaller amounts and use them up quickly. This also avoids rancidity. The serious olive oil user will have three or four different bottles open in the kitchen at any one time and probably just one in the store cupboard.

There is no point in keeping olive oil for more than a year as the next harvest may produce much better oil than the last one. Do allow yourself to appreciate the blessing of its continuity.

BASICS

Although this book is not a cookbook it is perhaps helpful to look at the basic uses of oil in the Mediterranean diet. There are mountains of cookbooks on the market which will give you a great variety of recipes; our task is to sort out the very basic ones, from which all the others will emanate—vinaigrette, mayonnaise, marinade, pizza and pasta, and general cooking and baking.

Character

In the kitchen olive oil reigns as queen in spite of fierce competition from a cheaper, wider range of oils. Olive oil triumphs because it offers variety in taste, aroma and colour. Twenty harvests of sunflower seeds will make twenty more or less identical sunflower oils. With olives, as with grapes, the fruit is better some years than others so that there is an element of surprise and variety of taste and aroma with each harvest.

History of Salads

Olive oil is best known as 'salad oil' and we must turn to our cookery heritage to see why. The first record of a salad dates back as long ago as the late fourteenth century, at the court kitchens of Richard II. In 1699, John Evelyn published his cookery book *Acetaria* in which he waxed lyrical over salads. He recommended in 'sallets' the ingredients should be so well balanced 'they should fall into their places like to Notes in Music'. His salads must have been a joy to eat with nothing 'harsh or grating' and comprising 'certain esculent plants and roots to be eaten Raw or Green, Blanched or Candied'. He had high praise for salads 'intermingled and according to the season'.

John Evelyn's contemporary, author of the *English Housewife*, was Gervase Markham. He came to the conclusion that salads could be divided into four main groups—a single ingredient, a mixture, just a table decoration or one which was a table decoration which could also be eaten. Between them, these two late-seventeenth century cooks made English salads into a popular dish. What happened to salad in the next three hundred years is a mystery, as it is still struggling for a regular place on the UK table. Could it be that olive oil was such a scarcity and so expensive that the dressing of salads (which is so important) was neglected?

Salad Oil

Even though olive oil was known as just 'salad oil' or 'sweet salad oil' for centuries (Mrs Beeton called it by this name), it was sometimes known as 'light salad oil' too. This is because an olive oil which is too robust with a strong taste and aroma is the death of a subtle salad.

Lettuce

Lettuce, a favourite basic salad ingredient, has a delicate taste. In this country, it was introduced in Tudor times and was praised not just for salads but for its nutritional value and as an aid to digestion and sleep. It was (and still is) valued as an appetiser, but its versatility means it can be served with other vegetables and fruits as a starter, between courses, with courses or at the end of a meal. It also makes a refreshing snack.

Dressings

The nature of salad requires it to have a dressing of some kind as it helps to moisten ingredients which are too difficult to chew without it. A dressing makes salad refreshing, lightens it and brings out the flavour of the ingredients and the personality of their particular combination.

The basis of most salad dressings is oil, which easily coats the ingredients whether they are raw or cooked vegetables, raw fruit or cooked pulses. Until the arrival of other liquid cooking oils to replace butter, lard and margarine, olive oil was *the* salad oil. Nowadays we have more choice as trade with other countries has become so much easier. In olive-producing areas, olive oil is still the premier oil for cooking and dressing salads. In the UK it now has a larger niche than it did and a growing share of the market.

Because of its roots in Mediterranean food, we must turn to the classic recipes of Italy, Spain and France to appreciate olive oil's place in the kitchen. From these we can give it a place in ours. Perhaps there has always been a place for it; isn't it just that we have not filled it before?

CLASSIC RECIPES

Classic Vinaigrette

The favourite dressing for salad worldwide is vinaigrette. In its simplest form it comprises Extra Virgin olive oil, vinegar and seasoning—exactly how much oil and vinegar is up to the skill of the cook. The recipe is merely a guide.

Oil

Choose an oil that will suit the salad. John Evelyn recommended that it should be 'light and pleasant upon the tongue'. Extra Virgin first (cold) pressing olive oil is ideal. Taste it before you use it as this can give an indication of how light-handed to be with the vinegar.

Vinegar

The trick is now to choose and add the vinegar to suit the oil. Malt vinegar will not do as it is too sharp; it is only used for dressing by the truly desperate cook. White or red wine vinegar is the classic choice. Cider vinegar will do at a pinch, but is inclined to be a little tart. Bear in mind, at this stage, that we are only discussing the classic recipes. Adventures with more exotic vinegars and additions lie ahead!

A basic three parts olive oil to one part vinegar is a good starting point. Shake them up in a screwtop jar to combine, and taste it. Does it need more vinegar or more oil? Adjust by adding more of one or the other. Then guess the amount of salt and freshly ground black pepper. Add these, shake again and taste again. Adjust seasoning if required and the vinaigrette is ready.

Vinegar Varieties

Now for the variations. You will find a range of vinegars at the supermarket and delicatessen: fruit vinegars such as raspberry, balsamic (best used by the drop rather than the

66

spoonful and blended with wine vinegar) and several vinegars which have been flavoured with herbs—tarragon, garlic, basil, oregano, rosemary, and so on, by steeping. The latter have the advantage of a more subtle all-round flavour of the herb than merely the fresh herb chopped and put in with the salad. They can all be made easily at home.

For a salad with plain cooked chicken try a fruit vinegar, and with cold lamb either rosemary or garlic vinegar can be delightful. Basil and oregano flavoured vinegar will often go well with a salad to eat with pasta.

Vinaigrette Variations

Apart from different-flavoured vinegars, sugars, fresh herbs, onion, cream, hard-boiled eggs, crumbled cheese and mustard can be added to give variety.

English mustard will probably have wheat flour in it and be very hot. The milder French Dijon mustard is more suited to vinaigrette and will not have been thickened with wheat. It can be bought in the UK but look for genuine French and not an imitation.

Vinaigrette à la Moutarde

In a cold basin or large cup, stir 1 scant teaspoon made French Dijon mustard with salt and freshly ground black pepper and 2 tablespoons wine vinegar. Gradually add the Extra Virgin olive oil, whisking with a wire whisk. (This is a better way to make it than shaking it up in a jar, as the mustard does not blend easily with the oil and the seasoning tends to amalgamate with the mustard only.)

Mustard Vinaigrette

Use the previous recipe but substitute ½ level teaspoon dry English mustard for the French. Make the mustard with 1 teaspoon water.

Vinaigrette with Herbs

Make a basic vinaigrette with 1 tablespoon wine vinegar, 3 tablespoons Extra Virgin olive oil and 1 level tablespoon finely chopped fresh herbs. Favourites are: mint, tarragon, thyme, lemon thyme, basil, chives, marjoram, broad-leafed parsley. If you want to use English curled parsley, use slightly less as the flavour is strong. This kind of vinaigrette is really for people with a herb garden or windowsill pots; ideally the herbs should be freshly picked. Supermarket herbs or those which have been picked for some time are generally not as good. Dried herbs are really best in hot foods.

Vinaigrette with Garlic

There are three ways of making this, from subtle to strong. For the subtle way, put 2 teaspoons Extra Virgin olive oil into a salad bowl with a sprinkle of salt. Cut a clove of garlic in half and with the two cut faces rub the oil and salt all over the middle of the bowl. Put in the salad (usually two or three kinds of torn lettuce) and finish the dressing with oil and vinegar vinaigrette.

The second way to make it is to use vinegar in which garlic has been steeped. The third way is to crush half a clove of garlic into the vinaigrette and stir well. This is quite a powerful flavour. Use it to dress a crisp and robust Italian salad with dark green or red lettuce, green and red peppers, sliced courgettes and tomatoes.

Classic Oil and Lemon Dressing

This is traditionally served with fish as it is a more subtle dressing than oil and vinegar. Use a screwtop jar and shake up 3 tablespoons Extra Virgin olive oil and 1 tablespoon fresh lemon juice, salt and freshly ground black pepper. Shake to blend them and taste. Adjust by adding either oil or lemon juice. Good served with chicken, white fish and shellfish. Variation: add ½ teaspoon castor sugar before shaking.

Classic Mayonnaise

No other nation is addicted to sauces like the French. Flour and butter roux with milk and cream form the basis of many classic hot sauces, but for a cold dish the cold, cooked flour sauce is not successful; so, a basic mixture of egg and oil plus vinegar or lemon juice and dressing is used to make mayonnaise. This is used for dressing cold fish, seafood, potato, hard-boiled eggs and coleslaw. For the cook, mayonnaise can be an elusive success as so many things can go wrong. The one thing that cannot be done without is time. Olive oil added too quickly will separate out from the egg yolk or curdle. Room temperature for all ingredients (and even the mixing bowl) is essential so items stored in the fridge need to be allowed to regain room temperature for a couple of hours. The olive oil needs to be measured out into a jug with a lip or spout for easy and slow pouring. (The electric mixer or blender would seem to be a godsend when making mayonnaise but too often the fine, instant control of the wire hand whisk is preferable.)

To make ½ pint (300 ml) by hand, use all ingredients at room temperature.

2 egg yolks
3 pinches salt
½ teaspoon dry mustard
1 tablespoon white wine
    vinegar or lemon juice
½ pint (300 ml) Extra
    Virgin olive oil (with a
delicate taste and
    aroma)
freshly ground black
    pepper
1 tablespoon boiling
    water (optional)

Put the egg yolks into a large basin and whisk for about two minutes, by which time they should make a smooth paste. Put in the salt, mustard and tablespoon of wine vinegar or lemon juice. Beat for another minute. Keep beating while you add the oil drop by drop until half has been absorbed. Relax a little with the remainder by adding it at about a tablespoonful at a time, beating it in and adding more. (If the mayonnaise is too thick at this stage you may add more of the vinegar or lemon juice and beat it in.) Adjust salt and add freshly ground pepper to taste.

If the mayonnaise is not going to be used immediately, beat in a tablespoon of boiling water to stop it curdling. Cover and store in the fridge but eat within a week. Serve with cold fish (especially salmon), hard-boiled eggs, prawns, scampi, salads with raw cabbage or brussels sprouts base.

HEALTH WARNING

Pregnant women, the sick, the young and the elderly are advised not to eat mayonnaise made with raw egg yolks as salmonella is a risk. Salmonella bacteria cannot multiply in a mayonnaise with an acidity level of more than 4.5 on the pH scale. A mayonnaise which contains plenty of vinegar is perfectly safe. Note that it is the egg yolks which present the risk, not the olive oil.

Mayonnaise Variations

Green Mayonnaise
Use only fresh herbs (not dried) for the recipe.

½ pint (300 ml) mayonnaise (made as above).

3 tablespoons each

chopped watercress and parsley.

½ tablespoon chopped chives

Blanch the herbs in a small amount of boiling water for two minutes. Strain and put into the blender with 2 tablespoons of the made mayonnaise. Blend and then stir into the remaining mayonnaise.

70

Serve with cold chicken or fish, hard-boiled eggs and vegetable salads (cooked, raw or a combination).

Lemon Mayonnaise
Make as for the classic mayonnaise but with the egg yolks put in the freshly grated rind of 1 lemon. (It must be whisked in right at the beginning.) Continue with the classic recipe. Excellent with cold white fish, chicken or hard-boiled eggs.

Lime Mayonnaise
Make as for classic mayonnaise, but whisk the finely grated rind of half a lime into the egg yolks when you begin. Good with prawns.

Curry Mayonnaise
Into the egg yolks, right at the beginning, blend 1 level teaspoon mild curry powder. Continue with classic recipe.

Cooked Egg Yolk Mayonnaise
There's nothing new about using hard-boiled egg yolks instead of the raw variety to make a creamy dressing. Cooks have been doing it for centuries. Here's an updated version of a recipe in Elza Acton's *Modern Cookery*, 1845.

2 egg yolks from hard-boiled eggs	1 teaspoon cold water
	1 tablespoon wine vinegar
3 pinches salt	6 tablespoons Extra
¼ teaspoon castor sugar	Virgin olive oil
small pinch cayenne pepper	

Mash the egg yolks to a smooth paste with the back of a wooden spoon. Add the salt, sugar, pepper and water. Mix well and add the vinegar. Lastly, put in the oil drop by drop from a jug, whisking it in after each drop is added.

Aiöli (garlic mayonnaise)
There is just one more classic recipe—aiöli, a garlic, oil and vinegar combination from the Provence region of France where, traditionally, it is served with cold fish and boiled potatoes. Use an old-fashioned wire whisk for best results. (Just two cloves of garlic are probably more acceptable to the UK palate.)

2–4 cloves garlic
¼ teaspoon salt
2 egg yolks
½ pint (300 ml) Extra
   Virgin olive oil

1 tablespoon lemon juice
   (freshly squeezed)
freshly ground black
   pepper

Peel the garlic and put through a garlic press into a pestle and mortar with the salt. Mix it with the pestle until it is a paste. Put in the egg yolks and whisk until they are smooth and the garlic paste is absorbed. Add the lemon juice and whisk again. Add the oil from a jug, a drop at a time, whisking to make it amalgamate. When half the oil is left be bolder in the amounts you gradually add. Should the aiöli turn out too thick it can be thinned down with the addition of a few drops of water or a little more lemon juice. Season to taste and serve with dips.

SALADS

You can see by all these dressings that salad can have far more importance than it enjoys at most tables. There is no point whatsoever in making a superb olive oil dressing if the basic salad it will adorn is not worthy of it.

The traditional UK salad is an unspeakable combination of tasteless 'flat' lettuce, tomato, cucumber and pickled beetroot. This is no excuse! We have a wider range of suitable salad vegetables than most countries, especially in winter. We could be famous for our salads if we just made more effort. Supermarkets and greengrocers have wonderful displays of vegetables and fruits for salad-making but few people buy regularly. The main stumbling block seems to be lack of adventure and kitchen education. Even really good cooks often fall down on what emerges onto the dining-table as salad.

Salad Ingredients
Here is a somewhat broader list of salad ingredients than our old friends flat lettuce, tomato, cucumber and pickled beetroot. One leaf, one root, one other, one fruit will make the basis of a good mixed salad.

BASIC UK SALAD INGREDIENTS

Roots Carrot, turnip, swede, raw beetroot (all finely grated), fennel, radishes.
Leaf. Lettuce (little gem, cos, crispheart and many other varieties), cabbage (red, white and green), young spinach, Brussels sprouts, watercress, mustard and cress, dandelion, lambs lettuce.
Stalks. Celery, spring onion, cauliflower, young broccoli.
Cooked Vegetables. Green beans, beetroot (without vinegar), asparagus, potato, leeks, cauliflower, broccoli, peas, asparagus.
Fruits. Sultanas, raisins, dried apricots, eating apple, dates, banana, avocado, tomato, cucumber, courgette, peppers (red, green, yellow), olives.
Herbs. Finely chopped mint, parsley, basil; garlic.
Cooked Pulses. Peas, haricot beans, borlotti beans, butter beans.
Garnishes. Toasted sesame seeds, croutons, chopped hard-boiled egg, crumbled or grated cheese, crumbled crisp bacon, toasted almond slivers, nasturtium flowers.

OLIVE OIL BREAD

Bread made with the addition of olive oil tends to have large holes in it and consequently have trouble rising. The texture is inclined to be rubbery and damp but that is its personality. It is usually given long proving times and baked with a dish of water on the floor of the oven. It is the ideal bread for tearing into pieces and using to mop up gravy, sauce or salad dressings.

FRYING

For frying the best grades of olive oil are not always required. Olive oil has a high smoke point; comparisons are lard 180°C, butter 110°C and olive oil 210°C.

Anyone who has a regard for their health will not be heard singing the praises of the deep fryer. A minimum of olive oil, to quickly fry meat or fish, followed by a thera-peutic drain on kitchen paper, is really the best of a bad job for this seductive, quick cooking method.

ROASTS, CASSEROLES, STEWS

Olive oil can be brushed on to joints instead of basting with butter or lard and used instead of other cooking oils to start off casseroles and stews. Too much oil will rise to the top and give an oily look to the finished dish, unappetising to people who are not used to it. Using a green coloured oil can be offputting for the uninitiated so probably the best colour for oil in this instance is the paler yellow sort.

OLIVE OIL CHIPS

The old-fashioned way to make chips, which can be dan-gerous due to a panful of boiling oil and leads to a fairly high uptake of fat in the potato, is quite unnecessary. Here is a new way which will produce crisp, golden chips with as little as 1 per cent olive oil.

Heat the oven at Gas 8/450°F/330°C and put a shelf near the top. Peel old potatoes and cut into chips. Put into a roasting tin and spoon in ONE TEASPOON of Extra Virgin olive oil per ½ lb (250 g) chips. Turn the chips over to distribute the oil and leave them arranged in a layer over the bottom of the tin. Bake in the top of the oven for about 25 minutes when they will be crisp and golden. Serve immediately.

Chips cooked in this way have half the calorie value of the deep fried variety. As olive oil is expensive, this is a much cheaper way to make them and a safer method.

BAKING

Olive oil is sometimes used for baking cakes and biscuits but is rather a strong-tasting oil for the more delicately flavoured egg, sugar and flour combination most people are used to. However, if spices and flavourings are strong enough it can be used for this kind of food. The oil gives a crisp finish to biscuits. The Spanish are particularly fond of this type of baking and have a tradition of baking for feast days.

PIZZA

Olive oil imparts a kind of light crispness to bread and pastry, quite different from other oils. The outer retaining edge of a genuine pizza is a good example. Forget the commercial variation of this centuries-old fast food which is usually thick and heavy-based with far too much fat. Instead, consider the real pizza which is a kind of flat, savoury tart—a thin layer of yeasted pastry with a raised edge to contain the light topping of fresh sauce, vegetables, a high protein food (sometimes) and herbs. Baked at a high temperature, the topping remains soft but the outer edge becomes crisp and golden. With a salad, pizza can make a good meal.

CRUDITÉS (DIPS)

There's no more delightful or unfussy way to enjoy a good olive oil dressing than with dips—little fingers or slices of crisp, raw vegetables for dipping in vinaigrette or mayonnaise. With their variety and bright colours they are an appetising as well as healthy start to a meal. Here is a list of what can be used:

fennel (sliced and separated into pieces)	cucumber (sticks)
	carrot (sticks)
spring onions	raw turnip (sticks)
radishes (sliced, made into sticks or flowers)	celery (sticks)
	cauliflower (florets)
courgettes (sticks)	tender broccoli (florets)
small tomatoes (as they are)	red, green and yellow
heart leaves of lettuce	peppers (part slices)

Good combinations are:
1 Radish, carrot, celery, fennel, courgette
2 Lettuce, tomato, carrot, radish, cauliflower
3 Cucumber, pepper, tomato, spring onion, carrot.

If serving individual portions, arrange the vegetables in a circle or fan with a little dish of vinaigrette or dressing. For a larger arrangement put the vegetables neatly in little mounds on a large platter with bowls of dressing in the centre. Vegetables should be fresh as a daisy and the dressing (vinaigrette, mayonnaise or aïoli) should be freshly made with Extra Virgin olive oil. Garnish with watercress, parsley and olives.

MARINADES

All round the coast of the Mediterranean countries small fishing boats catch the tide most days and bring back catches of shellfish, small and large fish. This is sold immediately and eaten fresh, the same day. Cooking is not elaborate—spit roasting or grilling over a wood fire. For the larger fish such as tuna and swordfish, which are inclined to be dry, a marinade can be used to keep the fish moist until cooked and also to tenderise it. Marinades are also used for lamb, beef and pork, especially for kebabs where skewers of meat are interspersed with vegetables and grilled. The marinade is used to brush over the food before and during the cooking. Any left over is usually spooned over the cooked food as a sauce so as not to waste the olive oil, but, if the cook has been too generous, this results in too oily a plate and even oilier food.

Here is a typical marinade: ¼ pint (150 ml) Extra Virgin or Virgin olive oil, 3 tablespoons freshly squeezed lemon juice, 1 tablespoon freshly chopped parsley or marjoram and salt and freshly ground black pepper to taste. This is shaken up in a screwtop jar or whisked lightly in a bowl. The oil and juice will separate out if it is left standing, so it needs combining every time it is used. Especially good on grilled lobster, prawns and any white fish inclined to be dry.

If using olive oil is new to you, you may like to try a blend of olive oil and sunflower oil. Try half and half to begin with and increase either of the oils to suit your taste. People used to the blander, rather tasteless oils will find this method an easier introduction to olive oil than using it full strength. Some supermarket chains have already thought of this and sell their own blends of olive oil and sunflower oil.

OLIVE OIL ON TOAST

Probably the best way of all (which happens to be the simplest) to enjoy a good olive oil is as follows. Take crusty, fresh French bread and cut it into thick slices at 45° to make long, oval slices instead of just rounds. Toast golden brown on both sides. Rub the cut part of a clove of garlic (halved) over one side of each slice. Drizzle with good Extra Virgin olive oil. Spread with a knife and sprinkle with a little sea salt (optional). Eat immediately while still warm.

Crostini

The Italian version of olive oil on toast is a little more showy. The untoasted bread is rubbed over with garlic on one side, the oil drizzled over and then they are baked in the oven or toasted over an open fire.

Brouchettes

These are crostini with a thick topping of cooked vegetables such as sweet peppers, raw chopped tomatoes with basil, olive paté and so on. They are served as a starter or snack and make excellent party food.

CHAPTER 7

Soaps, Cosmetics and Medicines

From the chemist's point of view, olive oil is a 'fixed liquid oil, pale yellow or greenish yellow' and (ever cautious as scientists should be) 'usually obtained by expressing the fruit of the olive tree'. It is insoluble in water, slightly soluble in alcohol but completely soluble in chloroform, ether and carbon bisulphite.

Olive oil is not a good detergent; a mixture of 75 per cent olive oil and 25 per cent coconut oil is considered better for ordinary toilet purposes.

The CTFA handbook states the fraction of olive oil 'as an occlusive skin conditioner, solvent and hair conditioner'. This makes it useful for shampoos, conditioners, tonics, hair dressings, cleansing, suntan and moisturising products.

By processing the oil, other ingredients can be produced for specific uses. The unsaponifiable and triglyceride fractions of olive husk oil can give a soft, waxy, solid by-product that can be used as a natural superfatting agent in toilet soaps. It is also useful in non-animal products as a substitute for lanolin.

If just the unsaponifiable fraction is used it produces an active moisturising oil which contains 65–75 per cent squalene, a key constituent of the lipids present in the surface of the skin. As a naturally derived plant oil, it is rapidly absorbed by the skin and makes a good emollient, hydrating and sebum-restoring oil which is compatible with all anionic and monionic emulsifiers. Used mainly for normalising dry skin conditions, the protection of delicate skins and the healing of wounded or damaged skin, it is obvious that it would be particularly suitable for babycare and sunscreen products as well as pharmaceutical ointments. It is a favoured ingredient in lipsticks and protective lip balms to prevent chapping in adverse weather conditions such as severe cold or hot sun.

Another important liquid (oily) derived from olive oil is a natural superfatting agent for syndets. It can be processed from the unsaponifiable fraction of olive oil and the triglyceride fraction of olive husk oil. It is used for shampoos, conditioners and liquid soaps, medicated and low irritancy soaps and pharmaceutical preparations such as douches and pessaries.

SOAPS AND SHAMPOOS

Before modern shampoos and conditioning agents, oil shampoos were based on sulphonated olive and castor-oil, containing unreacted oil. It is possible for olive oil to modify the foam structure of shampoos but in modern shampoo formulation is unlikely to give really good results. However, it does make a useful base for a mild neutral soap. When saponified with sodium hydroxide it produces a hard white soap called olive oil soap, Marseilles or Castile soap, as it was first produced in the Castile region of Spain. Because of this, 'Castile' is the name now applied to any white soap, irrespective of whether it contains only pure olive oil.

Two varieties of olive oil are used for making soaps. A cheap, household (or scrubbing) soap is made from green sulphur olive oil. It is called this unflattering name because the solvent used in its manufacture has a rather unpleasant smell. Only the better quality *golden to greenish yellow* olive oils are used for the manufacture of toilet soaps, although today they are more likely to be a mixture of olive oil and coconut oil rather than pure olive oil, due to its high cost.

Below are three typical old formulae for the universal hard, white soap we call toilet soap. Note they all use olive oil. Very soft with abundant persistent lather, fair to good cleansing properties. Very mild action on skin. Easy to make.

Castile Soap

	A	B	C
Olive oil	40 parts	30 parts	30 parts
Ground nut oil	30 parts	–	–
Cotton seed oil	–	30 parts	–
Tallow oil	30 parts	40 parts	–
Lard	–	–	30 parts
Palm kernel oil	–	–	40 parts

350–360 gals of Lye (KOH solution) per ton of olive oil

1   Oil in pan add 150 gals. lye 18 Tw boil 23 hours add salt to separate lye, rest 4–5 hours. Remove spent lye.
2   Add 100 gals. lye 32 Tw boil 4–5 hours, salt settle, draw off as before.
3   Add 110 gals. lye 42 Tw repeat as above.

French Liquid Soap
Liquid soaps for showering are by no means a modern idea. Here is an old formula with olive oil:

1	KOH	227 Kg
2	Water	minimum for solution
3	Olive oil	182 Kg
4	Palm oil	362 Kg
5	Coconut oil	362 Kg
6	Alcohol	170 litres
7	Water	5.6 litres

These raw materials were mixed and heated then thinned down with water until the correct consistency was reached.

Shaving Soap

Since the advent of the dry electric shaver, shaving soap use has declined as fewer men now use a razor. At one time shaving soap for the 'wet shave' was big business. Usually it was allowed to set in stubby-shaped sticks or in a shallow bowl which allowed generous lathering with a shaving brush. Lather creams came into vogue, and today shaving foams are available for the keen wet shaver. Here is a recipe from 1979.

Olive oil	2	Potassium hydroxide	1½
Coconut oil	6	Sodium hydroxide	1/3
Glycerin	4	Water	46
Stearic acid	38	Perfume as required	
Lecithin	2		

Mix ½ stearic acid with oils, put in double pan and heat. Add water and glycerin and stir well. When blended put in rest of stearic acid and other ingredients plus extra water if necessary, continue stirring, cool and leave to set.

Toothpaste

Combined with potassium hydroxide or triethanolamine, olive oil can produce an almost tasteless liquid soap which can be used for dentifrices—soaps for teeth. In formulae for this kind of product it appears as pulv.sapo, Cast. alba.

Shampoo

There are hundreds of shampoos available today, but it is only in the last two decades that there has been so much choice. Here's an olive oil shampoo formula published in 1933 (Belanger).

Coconut-Olive Shampoo

Cochin Coconut oil	30 lb
Olive oil	2 lb
90% Caustic Potash	8 lb
Water	22 pts

Saponify oils, stand overnight. Stir paste into 12 gallons of water till completely dissolved. Stand 8 days, draw off from bottom.

COSMETICS

The first use of olive oil in a cosmetic sense was to put it straight on to the skin and hair. It was particularly useful to the ancient Greeks who used it for massage to keep themselves in condition for athletics, dancing, games and war. Both the athletes and the dancers were a kind of entertainment at the games and the dancers performed at feasts as well as religious ceremonies. Muscle strains and stiffness were a constant problem, and olive oil would have helped to keep their bodies supple and prevent strain and injury.

Cold cream was first made and used as a skin cream by Galen in the second century AD. Some experts might argue that he stole the recipe from Hippocrates (460–370 BC), but as it is such a simple combination it may date back even farther: mix 1 pint of purified beeswax with 3–4 pints olive oil. Fresh rose petals were used to give the cream a delicate fragrance.

For centuries women have paid attention to their faces. Foundation cream provides a base to hold loose powder, giving a matt look to the skin. Modern foundations are liquid and tinted. This formula is as late as 1979 and is from a book for people such as pharmacists who wanted to make their own cosmetics. Note that olive oil is the largest constitutent.

Olive oil	125
Mineral oil	110
Ozokerite	2½
Carnauba Wax	13¾
Beeswax	20
Kaolin	100
Isopropylpalmitate	5
Titanium Dioxide	102¾
Perfume Oil	

Mix together by heating and stirring the first five ingredients. Then add the next three and blend well. Finally add perfume while cooking. Stand a day or two.

From the same book, *Make Your Own Cosmetics* by James Sholto Douglas, here is an afterbath lotion which is just a simple blend of five oils, including olive oil, and a perfume. Having removed a good deal of natural skin oil by vigorous bathing and use of strong soap, it is a good idea to put back the oil by rubbing in this lotion all over.

Almond oil	8
Sunflower oil	12
Groundnut oil	8
Olive oil	4
Wheatgerm or maize oil	4
Perfume oil	½–1

Mix well and keep in a closed container.

And from 1933, here is an oil to rub on baby's skin after the bath.

Antiseptic Baby Oil

Olive oil	4 oz
Chlorothymol	30 gr
Oil of Rose	30 mins
White Mineral oil	to make 24 oz

84

Do It Yourself Cosmetics

In the 1970s there was a vogue for making one's own cosmetics and toiletries at home. A rash of books appeared on the subject. One such book was *How to Make Your Own Herbal Cosmetics* by Liz Sanderson. As some formulae are as good today as they were hundreds of years ago, the author gave some examples. Here are two which have survived time without clinical trials. Would they have survived if they didn't work?

Anti-Freckle Cream
    Pumpkin Seed kernels
    Olive oil

Pound the pumpkin seed kernels into a powder. Add just enough olive oil to form a paste. This is an ancient recipe. Keeps the skin soft and removes freckles.

Dry Skin Treatment
This is an old recipe for dry skin. Beat one egg yolk into 1 pint of olive oil. Apply to skin and leave on for 20 minutes. Rinse off with lukewarm water.

Sun Tan Preparations

There is evidence that the Anglo-Saxons used tanning oil. The *Leech Book of Bald* gives this recipe:

> That all the body may be of a clear and glad and bright hue, take oil and dregs of old wine equally much, put them in a mortar, mingle well together and smear the body with this in the sun.

Liz Sanderson's book, mentioned above, gives two rather more appealing recipes for sun tan oils. Both can be made at home in your own kitchen. Make sure all your utensils and storage containers are scrupulously clean before you begin and measure out quantities exactly—no guessing. The paler colours of oil are preferable and will produce nicer looking cosmetics than the green oil.

Lavender Sun Oil
   40 g coconut oil
   40 g olive oil
    5 g essential oil of lavender

Shake together in a screwtop jar.

Sun-Oil for Sensitive Skins
   60 g sesame oil
   35 g olive oil
   a few drops Bergamot oil

Shake together in a screwtop jar.

Hair Treatments
This simple remedy is good for sea- and sun-damaged hair. Rub olive oil into the hair and cover with an old (clean) towel. Leave on as long as you can, up to six hours. Wash out thoroughly with shampoo and hair will be left shining and manageable.

Brilliantine
Using a hair oil to keep the hair flat to the head and shiny became fashionable in the early twentieth century. It was especially favoured in the '20s and '30s by Hollywood stars such as Fred Astaire and meant that his hair was as neat at the end of a dance routine as it was at the beginning. It went out of fashion with the younger generation in the '60s when the Beatles grew their hair and it became fashionable as a bob instead of the short military shaved look of the '40s and '50s.

Hair oil not only gives control to the hair but a shine. It was customary to put linen or cotton chairbacks over the backs of easy chairs and settees to protect the upholstery from such horrors as brilliantine on men's hair. This was in the days when many people bathed and washed their hair on average about once a week. Nowadays washing is much more frequent—sometimes twice a day (especially when showering). Brilliantined or hair-oiled heads were the bane of the housewife who was faced with greasy pillowcases on Mondays when she did her washing.

Here is a formula from as late as 1972. Notice that it is largely mineral oil with just a small amount of olive oil.

Mineral oil	99–80%
Olive oil	1–20%
Colour and Perfume	q s

(From *Cosmetics Science and Technology* by Balsam and Sagarin, 1972.)

Although not as widely used in cosmetics as it used to be, olive oil or its derivatives still feature today in skin creams, masks, soaps and products for the body, hair and nails. In the trade, olive oil for cosmetics is also known as Sweet Oil, Florence Oil and Lucca Oil. There are cheaper oils which can be used as a substitute, such as herring (minus the smell!), peanut or grapeseed oils. As some cosmetics such as lipbalms and lipsticks require an edible oil, the following can be substituted for olive oil: peanut, cottonseed, corn and refined rice oils.

Given the availability of cheaper substitutes, it is surprising that olive oil and its derivatives are still in use. However, its folkloric appeal should not be overlooked. With origins as a sacred oil from time immemorial, it still has a certain mystique. If it were not for the importance of its culinary uses, which tend to undermine its cachet in the cosmetic industry, it would possibly have held its place in this market, which at present is more inclined to avocado oil which has a more exotic, luxury sound about it. But as the cosmetic industry is by nature a cyclical one, who knows when olive oil will come out top again?

MEDICINE

Olive oil has been used for centuries as a simple medicine. Taken by the spoonful it is used to alleviate constipation. Taken by the wine-glass it is revered as a tonic, and in parts of Italy it doubles as a medicinal breakfast. Olive oil warmed in a teaspoon and dripped into the ear is used to soften ear wax. In spite of effective commercial preparations formulated specially for this task, it is still a popular remedy today. Rubbing olive oil into the skin to counteract sunburn is another old-fashioned remedy that has survived.

Age-old complaints such as arthritis have been treated for centuries by massaging olive oil into the affected joints coupled with a diet that has plenty of celery and primrose leaves in salads. Massaging olive oil into the scalp has long been a remedy used to treat baldness and for earache a mixture of olive oil, castor oil, onion juice and honey all warmed together is an old-fashioned home remedy. Olive oil to soften the skin and prevent wrinkles was widely used until the 1950s when the skin cream market took off. (Marilyn Monroe, who had a good skin, was said to have used olive oil in preference to expensive cosmetic creams.)

The Concise Household Encyclopaedia, an illustrated dictionary in two large volumes, edited by Sir J. A. Hammerton and published in the 1940s, sang the praises of olive oil even more loudly:

It is a valuable food and is also a mild aperient. For people who suffer from mild constipation, a table-

spoon taken every night will often prove most beneficial. As an enema it is very useful for constipation
with the presence of hardened faeces in the bowel.
Large quantities are sometimes given to people suf-
fering from gall stones. For burns and scalds olive oil
is one of the best remedies for immediate use when
the skin is not broken.

However, one of the most ardent olive oil fans of all time
was the Reverend William Martin Truder who, at the turn
of the eighteenth century, published a modest but ener-
getic tome, *The English Olive Tree*, or 'A treatise on the
use of oil and the warm bath with miscellaneous remarks
on the prevention and cure of various diseases, Gout,
Rheumatism, Diabetes etc.' In today's terms it was a
best-seller and by 1802 was in its second edition. (It
must have been popular to stay in print at the high price
of 5/-.)
The Reverend Mr Truder regarded olive oil as the
ultimate panacea. He was obsessed with it and lost no
opportunity to sing its praises. Here he is on the subject of
olive oil for anointing the body:

The ancients anointed themselves with oil to heighten
the comeliness of their persons and they did well for if
the natural diffusion of gelatinous juices (extracted
from the aliment and brought forward through the
capillary arteries to the terral parts of the body) be
wanting in general in weak and aged people what
better substitute can there be than oil outwardly
applied? The parched and shrivelled skin of the aged
and infirm especially those emaciated by sickness or
evacuations seems to demand oleaginous applications
for the powers of absorption are greater in these than
in the young and healthy.

A more vigorous approach than anointing he called 'friction'. He believed it was 'less conclusive to strong and general health than the daily exercise of running or riding to the point of fatigue'. He advised friction with a little olive oil in the morning and at night after a fit of gout or rheumatism, cheerfully adding that if continued as a custom it would probably prevent a return of the disease. 'Friction agitates the nerves and loosens them from that morbid adhesion to the vessels that constitute palsy.'

He recommended olive oil for headaches, bruises and contusions, pliancy of the muscles, smallpox, pleurisy, troublesome coughs and yellow fever. He also believed it was an extremely good insect repellent. 'No fly will touch venison or any other meat if rubbed over with the finest salad oil.' (By 'salad oil' he meant olive oil.)

Truder had a keen sympathiser in a certain Count Leopold de Berchtold who in 1897 published a pamphlet in Vienna advocating olive oil as a preventative and a cure for the plague.

> Immediately after a person is infected he must be put in a close room and near a brazier of hot coals, be very briskly rubbed with a sponge dipped in warm olive oil in order to produce a profuse sweat. A pint of oil is enough for one inunction. Operation repeated once a day till symptoms of recovery appear. Person who rubs patient should anoint himself with oil before beginning. There is no instance of anointers catching infection after a 5 year study.

As a treatment for the plague olive oil has had a mixed review. In October 1348 the Medical Faculty of Paris compiled a report which listed all kinds of food that should not be eaten in times of plague. On the subject of olive oil it was emphatic—'Olive oil, as an article of food, is fatal'.

Count Leopold was not above stealing other people's thunder to put across the olive oil message. 1900 finds him adding an unrelated preface to an essay on the Prevention and Cure of Hydrophobia presented to the Bath and West of England Society by an A. Fothergill. It was about the efficacy of olive oil, particularly in the case of rabies. The cure seems to have been a kind of egg and oil custard, a sort of hot mayonnaise. Not just the person who had been bitten but also the dog could benefit from his treatment.

Smallpox and pleurisy were two more scourges the Count notched up as curable with olive oil. His wild claims made the Reverend Mr Truder's seem modest by comparison.

Oil used for bathing, shampoos, for softening the skin, for gout, rheumatism, headaches, constipation, baldness, tanning; for shaving soap and cosmetic creams; oil for curing rabies, yellow fever, smallpox and the plague. No remedy has been used for all these except one—that of olive oil. That it failed to cure the last four hasn't dented its reputation at all. But do we know for certain it failed . . . ?

CHAPTER 8

Olive Oil for Other Uses

Olive oil has had many other uses—lighting, lubricants, heating, as a general purpose oil in countries where olives were cultivated and as a rare oil where they were not. Here are just a few of them.

LIGHTING

Lighting by olive oil only requires a heatproof receptacle and a wick of some kind. The wick is immersed in the oil except for one end, and when lit the flame is kept burning by the constant supply of oil drawn from the reservoir up to the light. More than one wick can be used if the reservoir is large enough—the ancient Greeks used as many as ten.

Being used to the harsh, cold and clear light of electricity it is hard to imagine what a pleasant light the oil lamp gives. It is not so dazzling or clear as electricity but is brighter than flickering firelight. If there is no draught the oil flame is steady and its light soft and gentle. Traditionally, in countries where the main fat available was from animals, wax candles were used, but where there was an abundance of olives, the oil lamp reigned supreme. Other, cheaper oils have now taken its place but mainly it has been superseded by paraffin and electricity—a more effective source but one which can never match the luminosity and flattering romance of the olive oil lamp.

Until petroleum was discovered in Pennsylvania in the nineteenth century, oil lamps burned vegetable oils such as rapeseed or olive oil. They were obviously better than candles, giving a steadier flame and more illumination. The tall glass chimney over a large reservoir of oil with a circular wick was developed in the late eighteenth century by Swiss-born Arni Argard. The open wick allowed air to rise through the centre with improved combustion and less smoke. However, it burned more oil and as it was expensive it meant only the well-off could use this type of lamp.

BOOT POLISH

Olive oil was sometimes used in Victorian times in the preparation of boot black, a liquid polish for boots and shoes, designed to give them a shiny appearance and protect them from decay and surface wear. In nearly all such products the base was a black colouring matter, commonly bone charcoal, mixed with substances which acquire a gloss by friction, such as sugar and oil. (It was this kind of blacking that the young Charles Dickens was employed in packing, when his stepfather sent him out to work at the tender age of 12.)

Spon's Workshop Receipts, published in 1909, gives a recipe for 'Cheap and good shoe blacking': to 1 lb best ivory black add 1 lb treacle, 8 tablespoons sweet (olive) oil, dissolve 1 oz gum Arabic in 2 quarts vinegar, with ¼ vitriol (sulphuric acid).

Paste blackings were also becoming fashionable, the forerunners of modern shoe polish. Most of these used cod liver oil and were expensive and 'put up in fancy tins' as opposed to paper which was much cheaper. However, there were cheaper versions made with olive oil. Spon gives the following formula: 2 lb ivory black, 1 lb molasses, ¼ lb olive oil, ¼ lb vitriol. These were mixed up with water to make the correct consistency.

The blackings were applied and then polished with a silk

rag for maximum effect, and helped to preserve the leather as well as to make boots and shoes waterproof.

CARBON PAPER

This was in principle like modern carbon paper, still used in duplicate books today. In 1909 it was called copying paper and *Spon's Workshop Receipts* gives the following formula: 10 parts lampblack, 10 parts olive oil, 2 parts ceresin wax, 20 parts petroleum ether.

The black and oil were rubbed together in a mortar and heated in a pan. The wax was melted in and after taking care to remove the pan from 'all fires and lights', the ether was added. The mixture was applied to hot paper which was then baked in the oven for 20 minutes to let the mixture thoroughly soak in. It was then hung up to cool. Prussian blue carbon paper could be made by adding that colour instead of lampblack.

This was an extremely dangerous item to make on account of the ether which is highly inflammable, and it shows the energy and courage people enjoyed in those days in making things for themselves, for it was included in a book written for the amateur and professional alike.

LUBRICATING OILS

For centuries, one of the traditional oils for house clocks was olive oil. According to *Spon's Workshop Receipts*, it was applied with a four-inch long pin flattened out to make an 'oiler'. The point was used to oil the mechanical parts that required it.

For oiling watches a small sewing needle fitted into a piece of brass wire for a handle, filed down fine and slightly flattened at the point was used 'so as to take up a minute quantity of olive oil'. When oiling clocks and watches, the distribution and application of the oil are important. Too much can increase the weight of the clock parts, so oiling requires expertise or the timepieces will not keep good time.

Olive oil has not been used for many years; finer mineral oils are now used instead. (Sotheby's London clock department were not impressed by Spon's recommendation to use olive oil which is a heavy, sticky oil, and doubted if it was widely used in the past.)

The heaviness of the olive oil was counteracted by mineral oil to make motor lubricant earlier this century. Proportions were usually 25 per cent olive oil to 75 per cent mineral oil.

OTHER INDUSTRIAL USES

A special potash olive oil soap can be made for use in the textile industry which needs to wash cloth when it is finished. As the oil is now so expensive it is only used on the most highly priced fabrics and cloths.

ANOINTING OIL

Anointing the body with olive oil is a very old and sacred ritual used from earliest times. It comes down the ages as a simple act and is still used in many different religions throughout the world. Usually it is applied to the head, but in some rituals and ceremonies it is applied all over the body—head, cheeks, shoulders, chest, hands, knees and feet. It differs from water in that it leaves a shiny mark where it has been applied. Sometimes it is warmed slightly before use, often in a metal receptacle, over a candle flame.

Today, the Church of England uses three anointing oils—the oil of catechumens (baptism), the oil of confirma-

95

tion and ordination and the oil for anointing the sick. The oil of catechumens is just plain olive oil, but for confirmation and ordination a sacramental balsam of olive oil and a flower fragrance is used. Called the Sacred Chrism, it is a sweet-smelling oil and is used for special services. The oil for anointing the sick is again just plain olive oil and is quite likely to come from Sainsbury's or any other supermarket. This is because the source of the oil is unimportant. What does matter is the *consecrating* of the oil. This is done by a Bishop on Maundy Thursday every year. The olive oils and Sacred Chrism are poured into three special containers and blessed, then decanted into much smaller containers and taken away to be used during the year by the priests until the next consecration.

A WEAPON OF WAR

How to dispose of the enemy when they attack the city walls. Heat several cauldrons of olive oil to smoking point and pour over the battlements on to the assailants below. The best time to do this is when the maximum number are trying to scale a particular place on the walls. A wise commander will have a stock of oil ready for sieges. Rancid oil is perfectly acceptable and just as effective.

CHAPTER 9

History and Folklore

With a history dating back to around 3000 BC, it will be appreciated that the truth about the beginnings of olive oil is to some extent guesswork. The cultivation of the olive probably began in Egypt and Ethiopia and spread to Greece, North Africa, Cyprus, Syria and Arabia, Archaeological finds also point us to Palestine, Lebanon and Crete. By 600 BC it had been introduced to Italy from where it spread to Spain, France and Portugal.

Olive oil is mentioned in the Bible, the Koran and the sacred texts of other religions, in Egyptian hieroglyphics and in Greek and Latin literature. Depictions of the olive appear on pottery, coins and tomb decorations from the ancient world and in miniatures and paintings from the dawn of the Christian era. It was an important crop because of its many and varied uses. Apart from the oil derived from the fruit, the wood from the tree was used for its attractive appearance in religious buildings and the leaves were fed to animals or dried and used as a fuel or to make paper.

GREEK LEGEND AND HISTORY

The olive tree obviously meant a great deal to the ancient Greeks as it holds an important place in their mythology. The story of how Athens, having previously been called Kekrops, came to be renamed, revolved around a single olive tree.

Zeus, father of the gods, felt obliged to interfere in a

97

dispute between Athene and Poseidon over who should have patronage of a new city in ancient Greece. In his wisdom he decreed that it should be awarded to whichever one gave earth its greatest boon. Poseidon, god of the sea, struck the earth with his trident and instantly a magnificent horse appeared, symbolising all the manly qualities and the art of war. (As with most legends, different versions come down to us through time. Other versions suggest a spring rather than a horse.) Athene, who was goddess of wisdom, produced an olive tree representing peace, security and fruitfulness. The goddess was pronounced the winner, the city was named Athens in her honour and she became its particular deity. By coincidence, only the vine and the olive have been commercially successful in the area, which has many deep natural springs.

The Greek goddess of peace, Irene, is usually depicted with a cornucopia in one hand and an olive branch in the other, making a connection between the olive, a time of plenty, and peace.

The goddess Pallas Athene, later to be identified with the Roman Minerva, is usually depicted with a crown of olive leaves; the arrows of Hercules were made of olive wood. Athenian brides wore olive crowns or carried olive branches to ensure a fruitful marriage. The right to wear an olive crown was a mark of the highest distinction, especially by a servant in the Athenian state.

Aristaeus, son of Apollo, is credited with the invention of oil mills. Pliny, the writer, praised the placing of different herbs in pots of oil to obtain 'exquisite flavours'. This was an infinitely better idea than his recommendations for preserving olives in a mixture of quicklime and oak ashes! Fortunately for the Greek digestive system, he suggested soaking the treated olives in water for eight days with frequent changes of water.

The Olympic Games

The olive played a significant part in the original Olympic Games in ancient Greece. The victors were crowned not with gold but with a simple wreath of olive leaves. Originally the competitions were for men only and were mostly war-related—running, jumping, boxing, wrestling, javelin and discus throwing and chariot racing. Harmony of mind and body were of great importance as well as a superb physique, perfected by exercise and training.

Herodicus (fifth century BC) is now recognised as the first known sports physician. His most famous pupil was Hippocrates who, like his tutor, advocated the use of 'scientific' massage with olive oil for athletes.

The placing on the head of a fresh olive wreath was the ultimate honour. Olive trees were grown at the western end of the Temple of Zeus and cut by a young boy with a golden sickle to make the wreaths. The beauty of the perfect physique crowned in this simple way can only be imagined, but the exquisitely modelled statues of young men are our legacy and are to be seen in museums all over the world.

Burial Rituals

Beautiful painted vases from the fifth century BC depict the rituals of the ancient Greek funeral. Wealthy people underwent a lying in state where relatives and friends grieved and the tomb was adorned with sashes and *lekythoi*, the 'flowers of death'. These were vases of sweet-smelling olive oil which were shattered at the grave or put into the tomb for use in the next world. The custom of breaking small containers of olive oil at funerals still goes on today in Greece.

RELIGIOUS TEXTS

A rich source of references to olive oil is the Bible. There is
a reference to it in the Old Testament as a fuel for the lamp
in the Tabernacle (Ex. 27:20). Solomon bartered the oil in

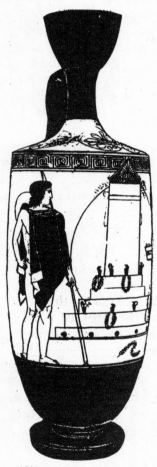

Greek lekythos *c*. 450 BC with a godlike youth (the dead man)
and a grave stele at the top of a staircase. Note the
lekythoi, small jars of olive oil, on the steps.

exchange for cedars and cypress wood (Kings 5:25). In times of God's favour the blessings of the land were 'grain, oil and wine'.

Olive oil in biblical times was valued for food, light and medicine and many other uses. It was applied to leather shields to keep them supple. To 'oil a shield' came to be an idiom for 'to make war'. It was used as an anointing oil. In Ecclesiastes, hope is expressed that people will never be short of freshly washed clothes and ointment for their heads. Olive oil is advocated for skin problems; for bruises, festering sores and even leprosy; for sore throats, earache, as an ointment, to improve the air and as a strengthening rub for skin and muscles.

'A land of milk and honey' conjures up a kind of paradise where there is no want—plenty to eat and drink and everything easily available. One of the biblical references to this desirable state is actually 'A land of milk and honey and *olive oil*'. Whether the olive oil brings it down to earth too much, or whether use of the Bible by people in countries where the olive is not a crop and has little meaning has led to the olive oil being dropped, is a matter for speculation.

The best known mention in the Bible of the olive tree probably occurs in the book of Genesis. Noah sent out birds to see if the floods had diminished. After two unsuccessful attempts a dove returned to the ark bearing proof that indeed the waters were receding—an olive leaf plucked from a tree.

The Koran also contains many references to olive oil, one in particular referring to the luminous quality of the oil. It illustrates the high regard in which the oil is held.

Charity and the Olive

The Mount of Olives is so called because of the prolific growth of olive trees in that area; so much oil flowed

101

that the gardens were called Gethsemane, a name derived from a Hebrew word *Gatshamanim* which means oil press.

The olives in biblical times were collected by beating them down with poles. The landowners were told that they should not go over the branches a second time but must leave any ungathered fruit for the poor (Deut. 24:20). This followed the pattern observed when bringing in the wheat harvest. Here the owners of the land were required to leave one corner of the field unharvested without gathering the gleanings. These were left for the poor as an act of charity.

For wheat this served two purposes. Firstly, the farmer did not want wheat grains to remain on his field as they were sure to propagate the following spring when he would be sowing a different crop on the land; and secondly, it was a way of providing for the poor who would otherwise have to beg for the harvested wheat. In the case of the olive it was a way of making sure all the fruit was removed from the trees and the ground, as well as providing olives for the poor and preventing the seeds from propagating.

This simple act of providing for the poor would be frowned on today. The farmer would be required to pay tax to the State on the whole harvest. The State would, at great cost, redistribute some of it to people required to prove their poverty. The gleanings would be wasted.

Agriculture

The oil had wide applications in the agriculture of the time since it was daubed onto fruit trees as a deterrent to pests, to insulate against frost and to reduce the worst effects of summer heat. Farmers also used it to hasten the ripening of figs and to keep ants and other harmful insects from attacking crops.

In the weaving of wool it was used to grease the fleece, enabling it to be more easily processed. It was also applied to the fingers of the weavers to soften them and make for greater dexterity.

Leather was rubbed with olive oil to render it soft and more pliable for the manufacture of sandals.

Methods of harvesting and extraction are also described: the olives were beaten down with poles, pounded to a pulp in mortars or with the feet and left to strain in wicker baskets from which lightest and finest oil ran off.

Anointing

The practice of anointing with oil was common in biblical times and was a mark of respect. It was made sweet-smelling by adding rosewater or other perfume. Jesus is recorded as rebuking Simon the Pharisee for omitting the act of inunction which was a civility observed during those times. The Apostle Mark records that Jesus had precious ointment poured onto his head and many books of the Old Testament refer to the practice of washing and anointing. Bear in mind that biblical lands were hot, dry and sunny. Oil for the skin and hair are essential to counteract the burning sun in such a climate.

ITALY

The first olive trees in Italy appeared somewhat later than in Greece. Initially they were a rarity and so few olives were harvested that in 249 BC a pound of oil sold for 15 pence—a great deal of money at that time. By 74 BC, less than two hundred years later, 1.25 pence would buy ten pounds of oil (about ⅛ of a penny per pound). As the olive tree became more widespread it only took another 25 years for Italy to be in a position to supply trees to neighbouring countries.

The olive and its oil were highly prized, especially by the Roman emperors as it was considered a luxury. On special occasions, such as the election of a new emperor, olive oil would be distributed as a precious gift to help the citizens celebrate. Olives often formed the first course at a Roman banquet (today, they survive as an appetiser), and eventually it was common practice to serve them at the end of a meal as well.

Olive oil was used by Roman citizens at the public baths as an emollient after bathing and drying. Slaves would carry it in a vessel when they accompanied their master or mistress to the baths. These had hot and cold plunge pools, swimming pools and steam baths.

At Pompeii, engulfed by ashes when Mount Vesuvius erupted in AD 79, bulging amphoras on the stone and marble shop counters held corn, oil and wine, three important staples in the diet. The town was quickly buried, leaving a legacy to be discovered—evidence of the use of olive oil in the kitchens, at the public baths, the market, the shops, the gladiators' quarters; in huge amphoras, in lamps, in small vessels. It was everywhere.

The Italians found several uses for olive branches. Placed over the door of a house, they believed they would ward off evil spirits. Before the use of coffins the dead were usually laid in the grave on a bed of olive leaves and then covered with more before final burial. In Venice an olive branch on the chimneypiece was believed to ward off lightning. In Rome there was a saying that wine within and oil without is the secret of health and happiness.

By the fourteenth century the olive tree had become so important that the punishment meted out to citizens of conquered cities was not death but the cutting down of their olive trees.

In some parts of Italy it is still customary to eat a mixture of cold lentils and olive oil on New Year's Eve, but no explanation is available other than 'it is the custom'. The meaning has been lost with time.

SPAIN

The Spanish believed that an olive branch hung in the home made the woman master in the house and that eating olives insured the husband's faithfulness. In some parts of the country the belief was held that the fruitfulness of olive trees was increased if they were tended by young children. If the olive gatherer was not faithful to his wife, a poor crop would result the following year.

EGYPT

There are several mentions of olive oil in ancient Egyptian writings. The Pharaoh Thutmosis III records that in every city where his men arrived they received good bread, olive oil, wine, honey and fruits. The same authority lists the harvest from one of his campaigns as grain, barley, green oil of olives, wine and fruits, and reports that oil was shipped to Egypt from Djahi. In the temple of Karnak, engraved on one of the walls, is the following, 'And the men of his majesty's army were anointed in Djahi with oil of olives day after day as is their wont during feast days in Egypt.'

LONGEVITY

Very old olive trees seem to have a special power. In Algeria there is an ancient tree into which pilgrims drive a nail to cure their ailments. A tree in Holly Street in Athens is believed to date back to the time of Plato and is proudly shown to tourists.

REGULATION

The first to regulate the olive oil trade were the Babylonians; after them it was the turn of the Phoenicians and then the Greeks. By the time the Romans were in control, special containers and ships had been developed just for olive oil. Imperial Rome decreed its subjects should pay their taxes in olive oil and there was free distribution and even a kind of olive oil stock exchange. There was absolute control by monopoly when the growing of olives in the provinces was banned.

The arrival of the barbarians put a stop to olive culture and for centuries after the fall of the Roman empire it was forgotten. But, as always, cultivation was restarted and the olive flourished again. The fortress farms and monasteries ensured that the tradition was continuous and after the twelfth century the tenant farmers took over the responsibility for producing oil. Today the EC has various subsidies and controls in all the European olive-producing areas.

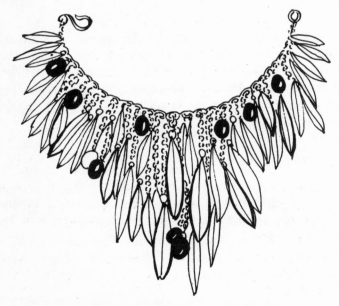

Necklace inspired by the olive tree by Taj Arpad 1994

SYMBOLS

In Imperial Rome the olive crown was worn by conquerors while in China it was the highest award for literary merit. The defeated in battle carried olive branches when they begged for peace and today an olive branch is still the sign for a wish for peace. Followers of Christ carried olive branches meaning 'I come in peace'. The olive or olive branch signifies not only peace but weather, food and strength. Anointing oils comprise olive oil and a fragrance symbolising strength and sweetness.

The dove has become a symbol of peace because it prefers to nest in olive trees, themselves symbols of peace; its peaceful act of bringing an olive leaf to Noah after a time of catastrophe also reinforces its symbolic image.

FERTILITY

On account of its ability to grow to a great age and keep on producing fruit, the olive tree became an ancient symbol of fertility. Assuming that peacetime is a more suitable time to be planting, cultivating and harvesting the olive tree, because of the number of years before the first crop, a stable society is essential.

MEDICINE FOLKLORE

God went to the Garden of Eden to see the patriarch Adam. He gave him a tree to plant in the Garden—an olive tree. Adam was told how to cultivate and tend the tree so that man would have the oil to heal his wounds and combat all ills. This example of folklore shows olive oil to be God-given. Adam is the gardener who ensures that the gift is passed on to man.

CHAPTER 10

The Cult of the Olive

Any visitor to Greece today who makes the pilgrimage to the ancient ruins of Delphi is confronted by the remains of fine buildings on a spectacular site. With the backdrop of towering cliffs formed by a great cleft, steep terraces and the bubbling sacred spring, it is as dramatic as any stage set. It is no wonder the god Apollo chose Delphi 'below the deep snows of Parnassus' for his first temple and the cult of the Oracle.

Now, as it has been for centuries, Delphi and its Oracle are merely ancient history. The mood of the once pagan holy place is difficult to sense as hordes of tourists scramble about the ruined buildings, snapping and filming their way from one curiosity to the next.

Anyone who turns away from Delphi to look down into the valley below will see evidence of another cult which *is* still flourishing—the cult of the olive. The valley broadens out into a flat plain, flanked by hills and sweeping away to the sea. Carpeting the valley floor are countless rows of olive trees, neatly planted and well tended, as far as the eye can see.

The two cults do have a link, for Apollo was a god of healing as well as order and reason. Olive oil is fast becoming a cult food for health and so for the olive it augurs well.

We have already seen how the Reverend Mr Truder and Count Berchtold made a cult of olive oil two hundred years ago. They were both high priests, as it were, essential in every cult. In Britain today there is one man who has done a great deal in the last ten years to promote the use of olive oil by generating interest and making supplies available. He could be regarded as a high priest in modern style. His name is Charles Carey and he commands respect from 'the trade' for his knowledge and enthusiasm. Undoubtedly, had it not been for his efforts, olive oil would not be in such a strong market position today. Charles Carey began to spread the word, and the oil, by travelling all over the country looking for new outlets, in a van carrying samples of single estate olive oils. It paid off, and today he runs a company distributing the very best oils in the country.

Talk to him about tasting and he will give the good advice, 'Look, smell, slurp and taste.' He will tell you that the belief that green oil is the best is a fallacy. His descriptions of tasting experiences and the range of olive oils now available are thought-provoking. When he speaks of the rising popularity of flavoured oils we know this is wisdom and we attend.

The cult of olive oil is a strong one because the industry is thriving and expanding, and olive oil is a tangible experience. Olive oil libations can be found in the supermarket temples and in the kitchens of followers. The sacred groves are in good heart and well tended in all the growing areas, this very moment. The silvery goddesses stand silently and patiently, producing the next harvest for the followers of the cult of good health.

*   *   *

Among the domestic olive trees, however, a crisis has begun. The family tradition is not as strong as it was, nor is the cult of the olive. Modern communications, transport and education have eroded the tightly-knit peasant communities and strong family ties. Families are more spread out and the younger members are not interested in gathering the olives—it is too much like hard work and they are not used to manual labour. They work in the towns and have the money to buy not just olive oil at the supermarket but American-style food and fast food. The few domestic trees that have provided for the family for generations are not so well tended. The trees need experienced husbandry to produce a good harvest, but only the old are interested or have that experience. When their generation has gone, who will look after the trees, plant new stock and gather the harvest? Skills will be lost as the continuity of know-ledge passed down from one generation to the next will come abruptly to a halt.

The economy of olive growing depends very much on cheap labour, just as the domestic trees depend on free labour. As the demand for olive oil increases, so do its costs. They cannot fall because it costs the same to produce a small amount as a large amount, litre for litre. When all the cheap labour has been utilised and mechanisation is the only alternative, the price will probably rise even higher to finance expensive equipment that is only used for a short time each year.

A rise in production will take years, even if new trees are planted. They will take a generation to produce a worth-while harvest. It is as if time for the olive tree moves at a different rate from the time measured by humans.

The Mediterranean-type diet came about by accident rather than design. Most people who enjoy it and its benefits are unaware of its value. Consequently as Wester-nisation of their diet takes place and it gradually moves away from the Mediterranean style, the low rate of chronic heart disease and long life expectancy previously experi-enced will also change. The rate of chronic heart disease is now going up as more animal fats, red meat and processed foods oust the fresh fruit and vegetables, fish and olive oil in the diet. The fact that the UK market for olive oil is expanding rapidly encourages olive oil producing countries to export oil normally used for themselves. Their loss is our gain but the price is in terms of health.

Soon after a baby is born it is washed—a simple ritual of acceptance into the human race. The rest of its life will involve very necessary washing with soap which is likely to contain olive oil or an olive oil by-product. Throughout life olive oil appears surreptitiously in toiletries, creams, lotions and potions, shampoos and conditioners for the hair and skin. It appears more obviously in food—salad dressings, soups, stews, casseroles, bread, biscuits and so on. When we die, part of the last ritual of life is being washed again, just as we were when we were born, with soap. So life comes full circle.

We cannot escape olive oil; it is part of the structure of our lives just as it was of our ancestors. Olive oil is in the shops, the kitchen, the restaurant, the canteen, the bathroom cupboard, on the table and in the medicine cupboard, and it is here to stay.

As time goes on, discoveries of its health benefits are backed more and more by science, adding to the legend. Now it stands boldly on the supermarket shelves in countries where the olive is not grown, gradually edging its way into the culture and fabric of society. The economies of countries where olive oil is produced are dependent on it and the olive oil trade is booming and expanding, helping to feed us well, look after our circulation and protecting our hearts. Long may it flourish and long may we benefit.

OLIVE OIL

Glossary

acid value: the number of milligrams of potassium hydroxide required to neutralise the free acids in 1 gram of oil.

aperient: another name for laxative.

aryballos: a globular flask with a narrow neck, used to hold oil.

axil: the upper angle between a leaf and the stem from which it springs or between branch and trunk of a tree.

Chorley Wood breadmaking process: a method developed by the British Baking Industries Research Association and still currently used for mass production of dough for bread which eliminates the slow fermentation process and allows the incorporation of increased quantities of water. This method of making bread on a large scale is suitable for widescale distribution by the limited network of main arterial roads in the UK. It has been largely responsible for the demise of the small baker baking several times a day on the premises. Some would say it has led to the decline in the standard of bread considered to be 'good', that can still be enjoyed all over the world where the Chorley Wood Breadmaking Process has not been adopted.

COMA: Committee on Medical Aspect. This is a Government Committee which reports from time to time on food policy.

CFTA Handbook: this is an American publication by the Cosmetic, Toiletries and Fragrances Association.

GLOSSARY

Degrees Twadell (°TW): an alternative scale for measuring the specific gravity of solutions by taking the first two digits to the right of the decimal point and multiplying by two, e.g. an SG of 1.4202 is equal to 84.04° Tw.

fixed liquid oil: refers to the volatility of oils which in this context fall into two classes—

1 fixed, which cannot be purified by normal distillation.

2 volatile, which can be purified by normal distillation. The method usually employed is steam distillation. Oils in this class often have strong odours and are widely used in perfumery.

hectare: surface area measurement equal to about 2.47 acres.

inunction: smearing or rubbing parts of the body with oil.

iodine value: the weight of iodine absorbed by 100 parts by weight of the oil. Since oils contain approximately the same range of fatty acids in different proportions, the ioidine value can be used as a guide to the degree of unsaturation.

lye: a solution of potassium or sodium hydroxide in water.

paraionic and non ionic emulsifiers: materials which help to form stable emulsions. They are complex molecules, one end of which is water soluble and the other oil soluble, drawing the immiscible halves of an emulsion together. The ionics have a positive or negative charge within their formula while non ionic are neutral.

peroxide value: the number of mille equivalents of oxygen taken up by 1000 grams of a fat or oil. It is used to measure rancidity. 1 mille equivalent of oxygen equals 16 mgms of oxygen.

saponification value: the number of milligrams of potassium hydroxide required to neutralise the fatty acids resulting from the complete hydrolysis of 1 gram of oil.

sebum: the oil secretion of glands distributed over the skin (sebacic glands) which help to lubricate skin and hair.

114

squalene: a hydrocarbon of formula C30 H50 which is highly unsaturated. The main source is from shark liver although it is also found in small quantities in the unsaponifiable matter of olive oil. It is a precursor of steroids.

strigil: a skin scraper (the forerunner of the modern squeegee) used by the ancient Greeks and Romans after bathing.

sulphonated oils: obtained when animal or vegetable oils are treated with sulphuric acid and then washed to remove excess acid. The acidic oil can be neutralised with caustic soda or ammonia.

syndet: an alternative (shortened) name for synthetic detergents.

trans fatty acids: one of two possible isomers of fatty acids known as cis and trans. The trans form has groups on opposite sides of the carbon chain

unsaponifiable fraction: that portion of the oil not broken down by reaction with potassium hydroxide solution. It comprises steroids, vitamins A and D and high molecular weight hydrocarbons.

References

Sirtori, C. R., Tremoli E., Gatti E. *et al*. (1986). Controlled Evaluation of fat intake in the Mediterranean Diet. Comparative evaluation of olive oil and corn oil on plasma lipids and platelets in high risk patients. In *Am. J. Clin. Nutr.*, 44/5 (635–642).

Mensink, R. P. and Katen, M. B. (1989). The effect of olive oil on total serum and high density lipo protein cholesterol in healthy volunteers. In *J. Clin. Nutr.*, 43/Supp 2 (43–48).

Trevisan *et al*. (1990). Consumption of olive oil, butter and vegetable oils and coronary heart disease risk factors. In *J. Am. Med. Assoc.*, 263/5 (688–692).

Buiatti, E., Palli, D., Decarli, A. *et al*. (1989). Case-controlled study of gastric cancer and diet in Italy. In *Int. J. Cancer*, 44/4 (611–616).

Moreira Varelo, O. (1989). The Diet in Spain. In *Europ. J. Clin. Nutr.*, 43/Supp 2 (83–89).

Mattson, F. H. (1989). A changing role for dietary mono-unsaturated fatty acids. In *J. Amer. Diet. Assoc.*, 89/3 (337–391).

Grundy, S. M., Bonanome, A. (1987). Workshop on M.U.F.A. In *Arteriosclerosis*, 7/6 (644-648).

Buzina, R. *et al*. (1991). *Ann. Nutr. Metab.*, 35/Supp 1 (32–40).

Katsouyanni, K. *et al*. (1991). Diet and Peripheral Arterial Occlusive Disease. In *Amer. J. Epidemiol.*, 133/1 (24–31).

Walsh, G. P. (1990). Dietary Change and Coronary Heart Disease. In *Med. Hypotheses*, 31/2 (135–139).

Linos, A. *et al.* (1991). The Effect of Olive Oil and Fish Consumption on Rheumatoid Arthritis. In *Scand. J. Rheumatol.*, 20/6 (419–426).

Wilhelm, G. (1993). Potential Effects of Nutrition Including Additives on Healthy and Arthritic Joints. 1. Basic Dietary Constituents. In *Z. Rheumatol.*, May–June, 52(3) 174–9.

Blauva, M., Boulton, P., Brostoff, J. (1984). Dept. of Immunology Middx. Hosp. Toxic Oil Syndrome. In *Clinical Allergy*, 14/2 (165–168).

Phelps, R. G., Fleischmaster, R. (1988). *J. Am. Acad. Dermatol.*, 18/2 1(313–324).

Bibliography

1 Hartmann, H. T. and P. C. Bougas. (1970). Olive Oil Production in Greece. In *Econ. Bot*, 24: 443.

2 Fedeli, E. (1977). Lipids of Olives. *Prog. Chem. Fats and Other Lipids*, 15:57.

3 Gracian, T. (1986). The chemistry and analysis of olive oil. In *Analysis and Characterization of Oils, Fats and Fat Products*, Boekennogen, H. A. (Ed) Inter Publ, a division of John Wiley & Sons, New York.

4 Fideli, E. and Jacine, G. (1971). Lipid Composition of Vegetable Oils. In *Advances in Lipid Research*, 9:335.

5 Kiritsakis, A. and P. Markakis (1984). Effect of olive collection regimen on olive oil quality. In *J. Sci. Food Agric.*, 35:677.

6 International Olive Oil Council meeting, 1985.

7 Diazani, M. V. (1978). La Persossidazione Lipidica Nella Patogenesi Delle Lesioni Cellulari. In *Simposio Su Il contenuto Ottimale di acido linoleico nell a dieta*, Sestri levante (Italia).

8 Babior, M. E. (1977). Oxygen Dependent Microbia Killing of Phagocytes. In *N. Eng. J. of Med.*, 298:659.

9 Vitale, J. J. and S. A. Broitman (1981). Lipids and immune function. In *Cancer Ros.*, 41:3706.

10 Harman, D. (1980). Free radical theory of aging; Effect of fat on lipid composition and function on the brain: 3rd International Congress on the Biological Value of Olive Oil, Chanea, Crete, Greece.

119

11 Viola, P. and M. Audosio (1987). Olive Oil and Health International Olive Oil Council, Madrid, Spain.
12 Ewald, C. A. and J. Boas (1989). Virchows, *Archives of Pathological Anatomy*, 104:271.
13 Taits, N. A. (1968). Use of Olive Oil in the treatment of ulcer patients. In *Urach Del*. 7:67.
14 Crawford, M. R. (1975). The role of essential fats in human maternal and infant nutrition with special reference to brain growth. 2nd International Congress on the Biological Value of Olive Oil Torremolinos (Spain).
15 Garg, A. *et al.* (1988). Comparison of a high carbohydrate diet with a high monounsaturated fat diet in patients with non insulin dependent diabetes mellitus. In *N. Eng. J. Medicine*, 319:829.
16 Ferro Luzzi, A. *et al.* (1984). Changing the Mediterranean Diet: Effect on Blood Lipids. In *Am. J. Clin. Nutr.* 40:1027.
17 WHO Annual Statistical Yearbook (1988).
18 Mancini, M., P. Rubba and P. Strazzulto (1985). Consumo di olio di oliva e regolozione della pressione arteriosie. *I. Congr. Naz. Terapia Roma* (Italia).
19 Ridgeway, J. (1991). *Taste and Flavour in Olive Oil*.

120

Index

INDEX